The Histology Handbook

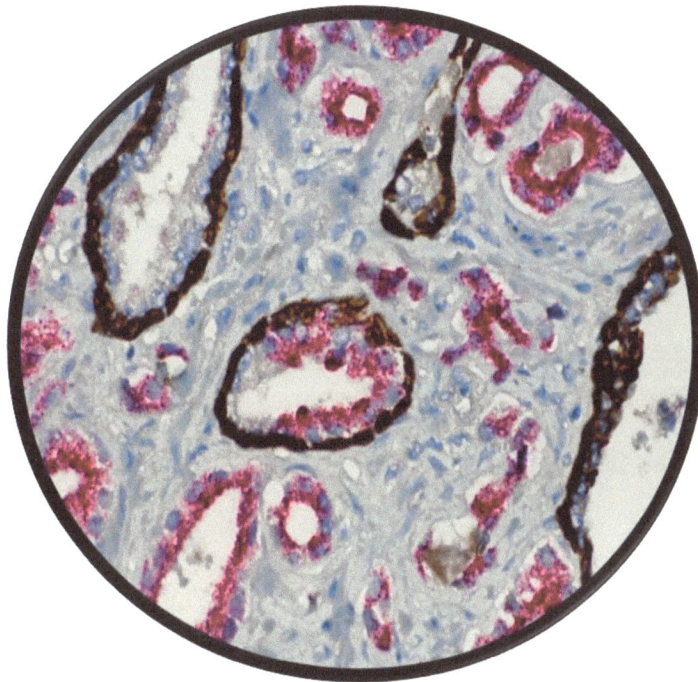

Clifford M. Chapman

The Histology Handbook

Clifford M. Chapman, MS, HTL (ASCP), QIHC

Copyright 2017

For additional information, please contact the author at:
Email cmchapman100@gmail.com
Telephone   617-957-8679

ISBN-13: 978-0692912164
ISBN-10: 0692912169

The Histology Handbook

Table of Contents

Preface

My entry into the field of histology was in the year 1976, the Bicentennial birthday year of our United States. It was, indeed, quite by accident; as I am sure many of you reading this have experienced the same introduction to our beloved field.

As a young researcher, with an even younger family to take care of, I had to learn and utilize histology procedures as a prelude to the final studies to be done using electron microscopy. Thus began my journey learning about the theories and performance of the myriads of histology tasks and stains which form the basis of histotechnology. These experiences automatically resulted in many instances of having to "troubleshoot" procedures that went awry.

Learning, carrying out and troubleshooting histology related issues for over forty years has had a positive side effect of generating a mass of histology related information – most of which has been retained inside my head. I have chosen to try to record as much of this information as possible in this current work, to allow others to have access to it. But what to call it?

A simple visit to the "world wide web" solved this dilemma for me. This work is titled: *The Histology Handbook*, as defined by the Merriam-Webster dictionary:

"Handbook: A concise reference book covering a particular subject, capable of being conveniently carried as a ready reference."

Even though the days of carrying books around are almost over in terms of human evolution, my hope is that this book will find its way into the many histology laboratories that exist in hospitals, universities and private laboratories. Whether available on a shelf in the histology laboratory, or on the "world wide web", I hope the information contained in *The Histology Handbook* will provide the user with the understanding to assist in the performance and troubleshooting of histology related tasks and help us all succeed in our common pursuit of "the perfect slide".

Clifford M Chapman

Clifford M Chapman, MS, HTL (ASCP), QIHC

Acknowledgments

The author wishes to thank Dr. Terence J. Harrist for his professional guidance and personal friendship over the past forty years. He also would like to thank Cheryl Halloran, Phyllis Gilardi, Joan Morabito, Janice Farrell, Nancy and Emily Collins, Lorelei Margeson, Jean DesRosiers, Lorraine Duhamel, Sue Pines, Ann Costa, Marcia McMenimen, Gino and Frankie Mercado – some of the original employees of Pathology Services, Inc. (1983) - for their professional assistance and friendship over the same forty years. Additional thanks go to Dr. Anne Allan, Dr. Lisa Cohen, Ana-Maria Jojatu, Ramon Silva, Louis Penta, Sarah Michaud, Frank Colella, Denise Broadbent, Catherine Lee, Jean and Judy Plourde, Lisa and Jen Zagami, Ivone DaSilva and Maria Lucia DeOliviera, Haimenot Gonte, Karen Katchel, Bill Bunke, Hana Mahdi-Alame, Trish Alman, David Gobiel, David Chau, Bernie Aronofsky and Nathan Chapman– colleagues and friends of the author's more recent ventures. More thanks go to the vendor representatives, some of whom the author has known for well over thirty years: Gary Beck, Bill Lannon III, George Kennedy, Brian Hurley, Justin Brown, Walter Burns, Rob MacDougall, David Patterson, Dr. Franco Visinoni and David Prine. Final thanks go to Barbara Morey and Mike DuFault, the backbone of the Massachusetts Society for Histotechnology – MaSH - for over 30 years, whose invitations to speak at annual Symposia helped me to hone my teaching skills. My apologies if I have missed anyone. Every person's efforts, support and friendship – along with scores of other coworkers and colleagues - helped to make the writing of this book possible.

The author would be also like to acknowledge the love and support of his family throughout his career. A man is nothing without the love of a family surrounding him.

Dedication

This book is dedicated to:

My parents, Ruth and Clifford Chapman, who taught me the values of honesty, hard work and family life.

My mother in law, Jean (Butler) Halloran, who successfully raised a family as a single mother – long before it was considered acceptable and fashionable.

My wife, Sheila. Without her, I am certain I would have accomplished nothing worthwhile in my life.

The Histology Handbook

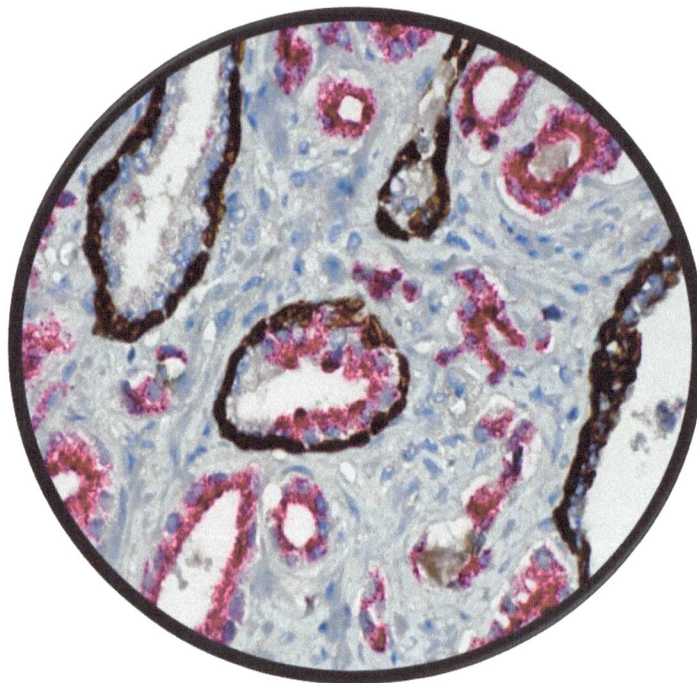

Clifford M. Chapman, MS, HTL (ASCP), QIHC

Histology Overview

In today's medical world, almost everyone talks about the most recent "scan" that they had at the hospital. These scanning devices make detailed pictures of internal body structures that cannot otherwise be seen without performing surgery.   CaT scans (computed tomography) use X-rays, MRI scans (magnetic resonance imaging) use a magnetic field and radio waves, ultrasound tests use sonic waves, and bone scans use radioactive markers to image and mark areas of interest in the patient. These scans can show abnormalities in patients, however, current methods in histology are often required to confirm specific diagnoses. This is necessary in order to determine the patient treatment and prognosis.

In histology what are we looking for in the final slide?

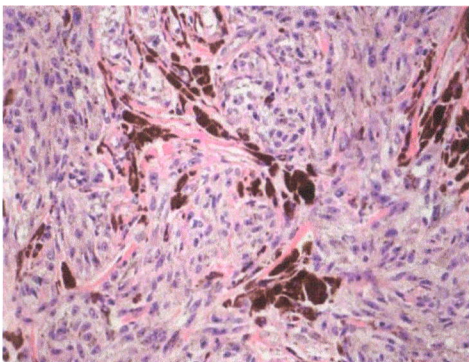

Figure 1. Malignant melanoma.
Spindle cell H&E
x 600

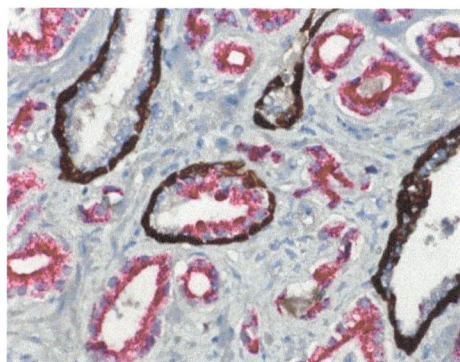

Figure 2. Prostate needle biopsy
PIN4 staining by IHC method
 x 600

Virtually every specimen that comes through the histology laboratory is routinely processed into a paraffin block, and a hematoxylin and eosin (H&E) slide is made. Pathologists are trained to render diagnoses by reviewing H&E slides. Even when frozen sections are made, at least one slide is stained with H&E.

Hematoxylin stains nuclei and nuclear material varying shades of blue, while eosin stains red blood cells and connective tissue varying shades of pink. The resulting tinctorial patterns are evaluated by a pathologist to render a diagnosis.

In Figure 1, a skin section shows malignant melanoma cells in a spindle cell form, including dark brown melanin deposition. If this original specimen was received as an excisional procedure, the surgical margins would have been inked during the surgical grossing procedure. In this way, the pathologist can also assess the surgical margins and advise the clinician as to whether more tissue must be removed from the patient. Malignant melanoma is a skin cancer that must be completely removed in order to cure the patient. Any malignant melanoma cells left behind in the patient may metastasize to other organs, ultimately causing the patient's death.

There are times when the H&E slide does not provide enough information to make a complete diagnosis. In these instances, additional procedures such as immunohistochemistry (IHC) need to be performed. While the H&E and other special stains rely on tinctorial results for evaluation, IHC uses specific antibodies to bind and localize specific proteins that may be present in the tissue section.

Figure 2 shows a section of prostate tissue from a prostate needle biopsy, in which the H&E slide did not show prostate cancer – but was suggestive of it. An IHC stain named "PIN 4" was performed, to show any "prostatic intraepithelial neoplasia" (PIN) and/or any prostate carcinoma. This stain utilizes a "cocktail" of different antibodies to demonstrate basal layers in the prostate (dark brown) along with any neoplastic and/or cancer cells (red chromogen). The abundance of red staining in the figure clearly demonstrates the presence of proteins that are made by prostate cancer cells.

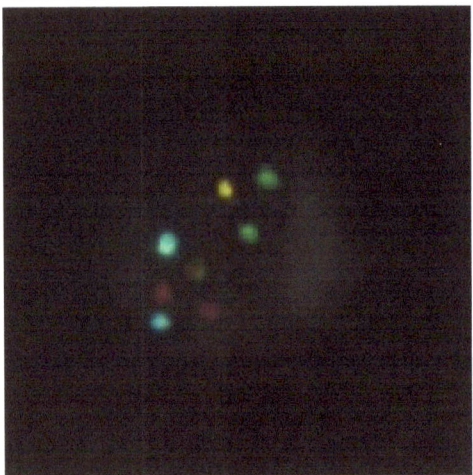

Figure 3A. FISH staining of malignant melanoma nucleus.

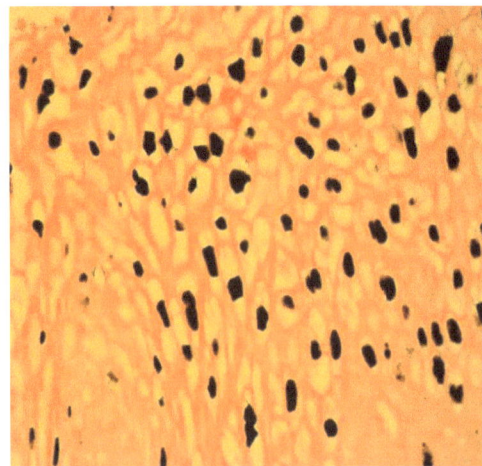

Figure 3B. mRNA staining for HPV

While IHC techniques use antibodies to localize specific proteins made by cells, the fluorescence in situ hybridization (FISH) procedure uses labelled probes to bind to specific sites within the nuclei of cells. Figure 3A shows one nucleus of a malignant melanoma cell binding four different colored probes. The probes are made to bind on specific DNA sequences on chromosomes. The probes are labelled with fluorescent tag molecules which fluorescence different colors when excited by different wavelengths of ultraviolet light. In this way, information can be obtained regarding the presence or absence of aberrant genes within the nucleus. This information can then be used to help establish specific diagnoses.

At the time of this publication, the most recent development related to in nucleic situ hybridization procedures is the use of probes to bind to single messenger RNA molecules (mRNA). Specific probes are used in conjunction with polymer based detection amplification chemistry to detect the desired target mRNA in formalin fixed paraffin embedded tissue sections. Thus, instead of detecting the proteins being made by a cell, this method can detect the mRNA being used to make the proteins (Fig 3B). This provides critical information about the cell one step earlier in the transcription process.

In summary, we can see that the histology laboratory has at its disposal an arsenal of routine and special procedures to probe the structure, function and genetic makeup of cells obtained from the human body. This information is vital in helping determine patient diagnoses, treatment, and ultimate prognosis. In addition, the use of proper surgical grossing techniques on dermatopathology specimens (i.e. inking of surgical margins) helps establish if all cancer cells have been removed, thereby helping to ensure patient survival.

Laboratory Safety

Histology laboratories contain dangers to laboratory personnel in the form of hazardous chemicals, biohazards and physical hazards. These dangers are minimized by identifying the sources and educating laboratory employees with regard to these sources and the protective equipment and procedures used to minimize and eliminate the dangers.

Engineering Controls

The first line of safety in the histology laboratory is the use of engineering controls. The histology laboratory should contain at least two fully functional, distinct air handling systems. The first provides heated/cooled conditioned air to maintain a constant range of temperature and humidity for employees and equipment to optimally function. The second system is an exhaust ventilation unit, consisting of an exhaust fan located on the roof of the building. This fan should operate continuously 24 hours, 7 days a week. It is attached via ductwork to all ventilated workstations and chemical fume hoods located in the laboratory space. Employees are instructed to use ventilated work stations when working with hazardous chemicals and biohazardous specimens. Additionally, there may be laminar flow hoods in the laboratory for use with biohazardous specimens.

Personal Protective Equipment

All laboratory personnel must be instructed in the proper use of personal protective equipment (PPE). This equipment includes, but is not limited to: safety glasses, safety goggles, face shields, non-latex gloves (i.e. nitrile), lab coats and/or impervious protective gowns, N95 respirators and half-face respirators with appropriate cartridges. The exact PPE required for each task is described via placard in each appropriate work station in the laboratory, as well as providing direct instruction to each laboratory employee. Each specific task in the laboratory must be assessed for potential safety impact, resulting in the specification of PPE for that task. All employees must comply by utilizing the specific PPE, which must be provided by the employer at no cost to the employee.

Safety Training

All laboratory employees must be given safety training upon initial assignment and annually thereafter. All employees are then required to review the laboratory safety manual annually. The laboratory safety manual must be available in the work area at all times. The laboratory safety manual should include sections on General Safety Policies, Fire Prevention/Disaster Plans, Chemical Hygiene Plan/Hazardous Materials/Formaldehyde Standard, Biohazard Policy/Bloodborne Pathogens, Accident First Aid/Reporting, Ergonomics, and Equipment Safety, at a minimum.

Safety Corner

There should be a source of everyday safety information and it is suggested to have a "Safety Corner" located in the laboratory. Pertinent safety information is posted for all employees and includes:
- Fire extinguisher operation – **PASS**
[**P**ull the safety pin / **A**im the nozzle at the base of the fire / **S**queeze the handle / **S**weep the base of the fire.]
- Fire Discovery procedure – **RACE**
[**R**escue / **A**ctivate Alarm / **C**onfine the Fire / **E**vacuate, Extinguish
- Evacuation map
- Disaster evacuation directions
- Chemical spill procedure
- MSDS binders / access to on line MSDS
- OSHA 300A log
- List of emergency contact numbers

General Safety Rules and Instructions

While all safety procedures are contained in the laboratory safety manual which all employees have access to, the following general safety rules are universally adopted and should be included in any and all safety instruction. All laboratory personnel are expected to be familiar with the following safety concepts.

1. There is no smoking in the laboratory or building.
2. There is no eating or drinking in the laboratory.
3. Every task in the laboratory has specific PPE designated to be used.

4. Any and all waste must be deposited in one of the following waste streams:
   - Chemical waste: waste drums are provided.
   - Biohazardous waste: double red bag biohazard containers are provided. All gloves are to be disposed of here.
   - Sharps waste: hard plastic sharps containers are provided.
   - Sanitary waste: regular trash barrels are provided.
5. All waste is properly manifested for legal disposal by licensed facilities.
6. Proper closed toe, rubber soled footwear must be worn in the laboratory.
7. Ventilated workstations must be used when handling chemicals and/or biohazardous materials.

In summary, it is the responsibility of the employer to provide safety training and PPE to laboratory personnel, and it is the laboratory employees' responsibility to use proper PPE and follow all safety procedures. That is the only way to guarantee everyone's safety while working in the laboratory.

The histology laboratory is a dangerous place to work for employees. Sharp knives, slick floors, hazardous chemicals and bloodborne pathogens are just the main sources of potential accidents. A way to keep histology laboratory employees safe is to provide information on dangers, explain the ways in which employees can protect themselves, and provide annual training to reinforce this information. This is not just a good plan. In most instances, this plan is backed by laws and regulations.

OSHA – The Formaldehyde Standard

Passed in December 1987, the standard protects all workers, laboratory and industrial alike. The standard was revised in May 1992 to incorporate lower exposure limits. Copies of the standard can be obtained from your local OSHA office, or on line.

OSHA uses different types of limits for airborne exposures, which reflect *Permissible Exposure Limits (PEL)*.

Time Weighted Average (TWA) is the airborne concentration averaged over eight consecutive hours. The TWA for formaldehyde is 0.75 ppm. No employee may be exposed to more than 0.75 ppm of formaldehyde over eight hours.

Short Term Exposure Limit (STEL) is the airborne concentration averaged over the worst 15 minutes. The STEL for formaldehyde is 2 ppm.

OSHA has also set an Action Level for formaldehyde of 0.5 ppm averaged over 8 hours. If this limit is reached or exceeded, the employee must be notified and steps taken immediately to adjust procedures that result in a decrease of the airborne concentration.

Employee monitoring is required to document the exposures existing in the laboratory. Initial monitoring of each exposed employee is required, unless monitoring has been done previously for a particular job description. Initial monitoring must be repeated if there is a change in work procedures or control systems. If an employee displays any exposure symptoms (i.e. respiratory, dermal, etc.) the employee must be monitored immediately.

If either the TWA or STEL is exceeded, the employer can:
- Install engineering controls, such as increased ventilation.
- Change work practice controls, such as procedural changes.
- Provide and require use of respirators.

Periodic employee monitoring depends on the initial monitoring results.
- If exposure levels are at or above the Action Level of 0.5 ppm, immediate monitoring must be done for each employee or job description and continued until the issue is resolved.
- If the STEL is exceeded, immediate monitoring must occur and continue until the issue is resolved.

Periodic monitoring may be discontinued if two successive samples taken at least seven days apart are below the Action Level and STEL.

Recommendation: In our laboratory, we monitor employees annually, even though the standard does not require it. We feel it is important for both employer and employee to make certain the work environment is safe for everyone.

Required: Safety goggles, gloves and an impervious gown, as well as access to an eyewash station and safety shower are required when handling formalin, regardless of the exposure limit (Figure 4).

Remember:

> ## CAUTION. CONTAINS FORMALDEHYDE.
> Toxic by inhalation and if swallowed. Irritating to the eyes, respiratory system, and skin. May cause sensitization by inhalation or by skin contact. Risk of serious damage to eyes. May cause cancer; repeated or prolonged exposure increases the risk.

The above label must be present on EVERY container and specimen bottle of formaldehyde. It is there for a reason. Formaldehyde is a POISON and CARCINOGEN. You must handle it with proper personal protective equipment (PPE) using a ventilated work station...always...without exception.

Histology laboratory personnel who change out tissue processors are especially prone to formaldehyde liquid and vapor exposure. Personnel must wear the PPE described above while handling formaldehyde. Additionally, when pouring containers of formaldehyde (i.e. from on board tissue processors, into waste containers), employees should be performing this function in a fume hood to prevent exposure. Alternatively, employees may be fit-tested for a respirator to wear during the handling of formaldehyde. Goggles, rather than safety glasses, are the eye protection of choice, since they protect against splashes and vapors (Figure 5).

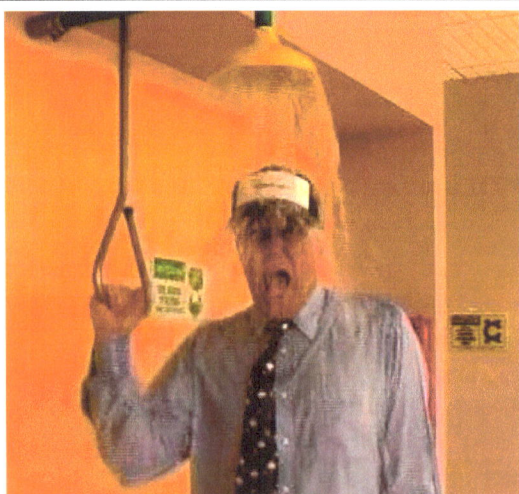

Figure 4. Safety shower in operation.

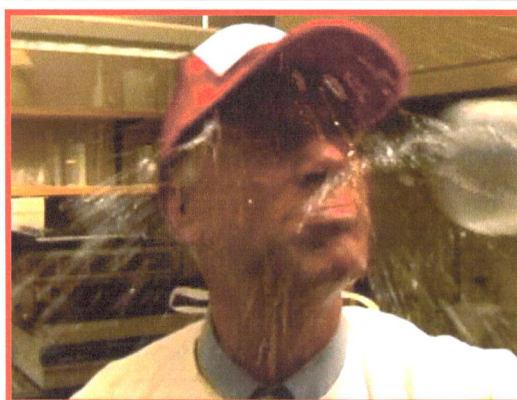

Figure 5. Accidental face splash, with no safety goggles.

Fume Hoods: The Front Line of Protection

All laboratory personnel should be aware of and know what personal protective equipment (PPE) they should wear while performing various tasks in the histology laboratory. Employers are responsible for educating laboratory personnel about what hazardous chemicals they might handle, how to handle them safely and what specific protective equipment to wear for each and every task that is performed in the laboratory.

Employers must make use of engineering controls to help protect workers as well. In addition to the usual heating and cooling system of the work area, the histology laboratory should also have workstations that are vented to the outside, or make use of filters if vented back to the inside air.

Usually, there is at least one chemical fume hood located in the laboratory vented to the outside. Employees can use this space to pour off flammable/noxious chemicals, coverslip, or perform special stains that may generate hazardous fumes (i.e. mixing hydrochloric acid with potassium ferrocyanide to make the working solution of the Gomori's stain for iron).

Performing the surgical grossing of specimens is one task that requires both full PPE and a ventilated work station. Laboratory employees must be protected against formaldehyde fumes and blood borne pathogens. Most pathology laboratories make use of units referred to as "grossing stations". The most common grossing station is made of stainless steel which comprises the work surface, sides and front. This accommodates ease of cleaning and disinfection. Plumbing and a sink may be included for applications where large specimens (i.e. whole organs, limbs, etc.) are received. Strong lighting is required as well. Generally, a grossing station has a series of small exhaust fans (usually four) situated at the back of the work surface. Since formaldehyde is heavier than air (i.e. vapor pressure = 1.1), these fans pull the formaldehyde vapors into the back of the station, where they are collected into one vertically rising duct. The vapors are propelled along the inside of the duct with extra fans to move the vapors up the ductwork, to the outside of the building. An important regulation is that the exhaust duct on the roof of the building must not be anywhere near any intake vents for the building ventilation. Figure 6 shows an example of such a grossing station.

Another grossing station uses side and downdraft principles to manage heavy formaldehyde fumes. Figure 7 shows how the intake fans pull the fumes sideways, and move then downward. Once propelled downward, the fumes can go through a filter system to remove the hazardous fumes. This clean air can now be moved back into the laboratory. Clearly, the filters must be changed on a regular basis, according to the manufacturer's recommendations. It is important to select the exact grossing station configuration that will work the best for your laboratory.

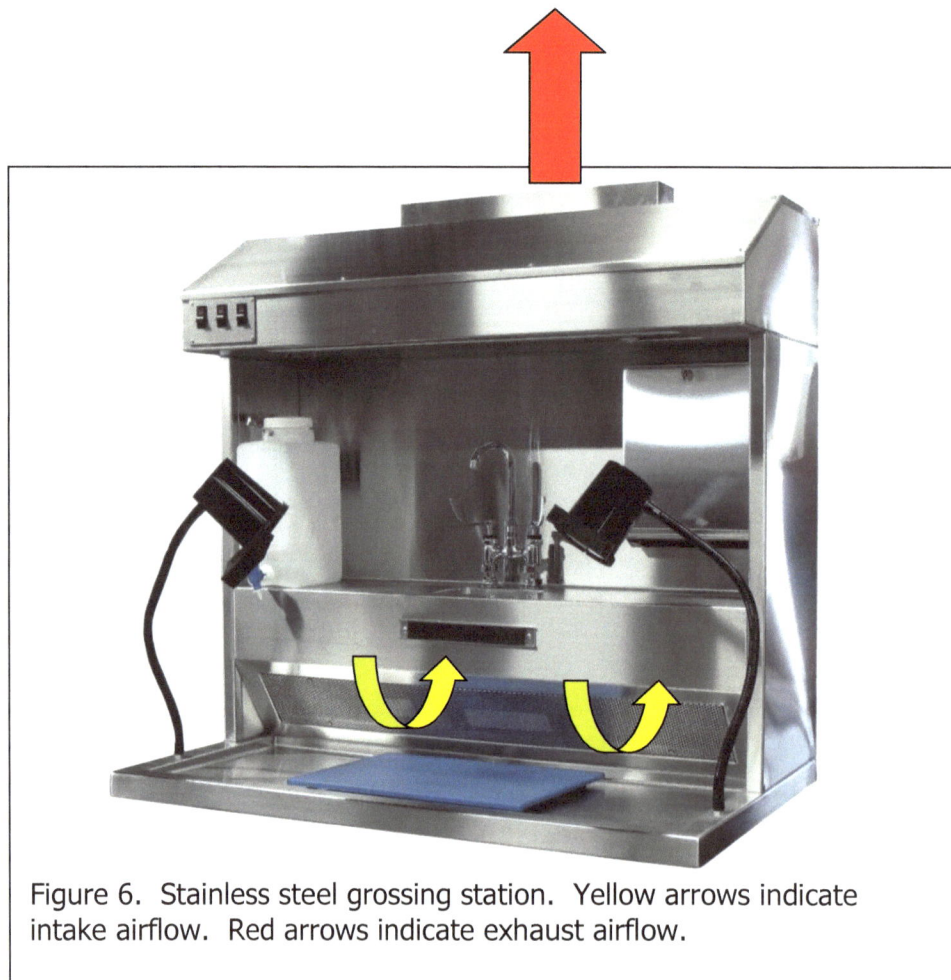

Figure 6. Stainless steel grossing station. Yellow arrows indicate intake airflow. Red arrows indicate exhaust airflow.

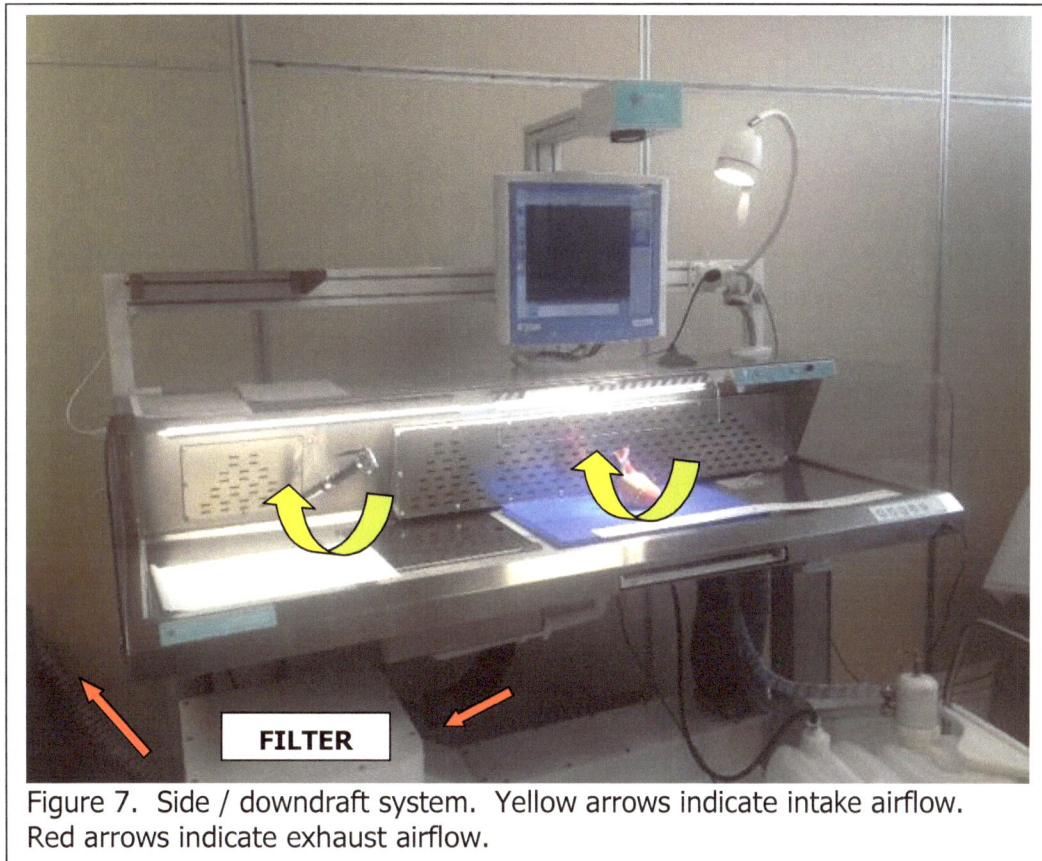

Figure 7. Side / downdraft system. Yellow arrows indicate intake airflow. Red arrows indicate exhaust airflow.

Rules and Regulations

OSHA passed "Occupational Exposure to Hazardous Chemicals in the Laboratory" in January 1990, which is known as the Laboratory Standard. It is to be used in conjunction with the Hazard Communication Standard and Chemical Hygiene Plan to inform and train employees on the dangers of exposure to hazardous chemicals that they may work with.

Chemical Hygiene Plan

Employers were required to write and implement a Chemical Hygiene Plan (CHP) by January 31, 1991. At a minimum, the CHP must describe work practices, procedures and policies to protect workers from hazardous chemicals. The following elements must be part of the CHP:

- Description of procedures and personal protective equipment (PPE) required to perform specific tasks.
- Description of specific exposure control methods.
- Description of methods used to confirm proper operation and function of mechanical controls (i.e. fume hoods, ventilation, etc.).
- Identification of any procedures hazardous enough to warrant prior approval by the employee before implementation.
- Description of employee training and medical consultations.
- Designation of a Chemical Hygiene Officer or Committee.
- Designation of an area within the laboratory where "select carcinogens" are handled.
- Description of procedures for the safe removal of contaminated waste, and decontamination procedures.

Hazard Communication Standard

This "Right to Know" standard was pre-empted by the Laboratory Standard. However, some aspects still apply.

- Material Safety Data Sheets (MSDS) for any hazardous chemical in the workplace must be on file, and available to employees. These are now known as "Safety Data Sheets" (SDS).
- Employers must have a written hazard communication program. Under the Laboratory Standard, the CHP takes its place. Note that the Formaldehyde and Bloodborne Pathogen Standards require their own written programs.
- Hazardous chemicals are required to be labeled with the identity of the chemical and the appropriate hazard warning.
- Employees must be provided with information and training upon initial assignment and whenever a new hazard is introduced.
- Employers must provide annual training and reviews.

Chemical Storage

The worst thing you can do in your laboratory is to store all the chemicals by alphabetical order. Each chemical has its own characteristics, detailed in the SDS that will determine the storage conditions. Additionally, the SDS should spell out what chemical incompatibilities exist- that is, what chemicals to ***not*** store it with.

Chemical Storage Considerations

Light sensitive chemicals must be stored in dark containers in dark, cool storage areas. Peroxides fall into this category, as do silver salts, dioxane, acetaldehyde, sodium iodide, mercuric chloride and mercuric iodide. (Note- you should not have any mercury compounds in your laboratory- see the *Mercury* section.)

Acids should be stored by themselves, in an acid cabinet away from formaldehyde, bases, alcohols and oxidizers.

Bleach is a base, composed of 5% sodium hypochlorite. If it is mixed with formaldehyde or ammonium hydroxide, toxic gases can be released. Bleach should also not be stored next to acids or methanol.

Flammable compounds such as acetone, xylene and alcohol should ***never*** be stored in a regular laboratory refrigerator or freezer. These chemicals can vaporize and leak from their containers, forming a mixture inside the refrigerator/freezer. Then, when ignited by a spark (i.e. the condenser unit coming on), they can explode. Flammables should be stored in a flammable cabinet, or in an approved explosion-proof refrigerator.

Carcinogens

Some chemicals are capable of causing alterations in the DNA (genetic material). Changes in the DNA can cause mutations, cancer and or reproductive damage. These chemicals are referred to as "carcinogens" and are covered separately under the laboratory standard. They must be kept in a secure and labeled area within the laboratory, and employees must handle them with extreme care, including use of personal protective equipment and proper ventilation. Current CAP regulations require all chemicals to be assessed for carcinogenicity, reproductive toxicity and acute hazards, as well. The following chemicals may be found in the histology laboratory and are considered carcinogens:

The following chemicals are carcinogens / hazardous to handle:

Arsenic   Crystal violet
Auramine O   DAB (diamino-benzidine)
Basic fuchsin/pararosaniline/basic red 9   Dimethyl formamide
Benzene   Dioxane
Benzidine based dyes   formaldehyde
Chlorazol black   lead compounds
Chloroform   nickel compounds
Chrome salts (chromic acid, K dichromate)   propylene oxide
Congo red   pyridine

[List taken from Laboratory Safety. NSH Self Assessment Booklet. 1st edition. page 33, 2004.]

Mercury
There is no need to keep any mercury compounds in the histology laboratory. There are many substitutes available today. Do the substitutes work as good as the original mercury compounds? Sometimes yes, sometimes no. Do the substitutes work well enough to produce optimal staining? Most certainly – yes.

You should dispose of your mercury thermometers and replace them with organic filled thermometers as well. Mercury is a very toxic poison, and has no place in today's histology laboratory.

Spills
Each laboratory should have specific instructions regarding what procedure to follow in the case of a chemical spill. Some laboratories located in a hospital setting may have a Safety Department to call in order to put the Hazardous Material (HAZMAT) cleanup crew on alert. Other smaller laboratories may have to rely on their own resources, or use an outside contractor. Whatever the situation, laboratory employees need to know what to do in case of a chemical spill. In addition, the procedure must be posted. A sample Spill Procedure follows.

In case of a spill:
(1) NOTIFY coworkers so that they may exit the area,
(2) CONTAIN the spill with absorbent from any of the spill control stations located in the laboratory, (if possible)
(3) NOTIFY the Chemical Hygiene Officer or Technician in charge so they may arrange for clean up.

Laboratory design can help this problem and provide a "safe haven" outside of the laboratory. Ideally, the laboratory space should be enclosed, with two exit doors that remain closed at all times. With the exhaust ventilation operating, this should make the laboratory "negative" with respect to the areas outside of the laboratory. That is, air should be moving into and through the laboratory at all times. Thus, in case of a spill that generates hazardous fumes, the "negative" laboratory space will protect the remainder of the adjoining spaces by preventing the diffusion of fumes outside of the laboratory.

Physical Hazards

Falls
Accidental falls are the number one threat to safety in the histology laboratory. Laboratory employees should not be at prime risk, as they are supposed to wear non-slip footwear. However, office staff and visitors are at a very high risk of slipping, falling and being injured. Many facilities have a carpeted office area.   Office staff becomes accustomed to the particular "coefficient of friction" between their footwear and the carpet. Then, when they enter the laboratory and step onto the tile floor, this coefficient of friction is very different, and their feet literally slip out from under them. It is similar to walking along a snow bank, and then stepping out onto ice. Falls can seriously injure the affected person. In order to minimize accidental falls, the following recommendations are made:

- Prohibit all non-laboratory personnel from entering the laboratory.
- If this cannot be done, mandate that all office staff and visitors into the laboratory wear non-slip footwear.
- A laboratory staff member should accompany any visitor entering the laboratory, to remind them to "walk easy" on the tile floor.

Cuts

Cuts are the second most common threat in the histology laboratory. Any histologist who is cutting blocks on a rotary microtome is at risk. While personnel are safer today with the use of disposable blades, there are several occasions when a histologist can get cut.

- Most disposable blades are provided in an injector type dispenser. When the blade is being dispensed, the histologist runs the risk of pushing the blade across an exposed finger.
- When the histologist removes or inserts a block into the microtome, it is imperative that the hand wheel is in the locked position. If the wheel is not locked, the downward force of working the chuck can move it downward, into the blade, causing a cut.
- When a histologist is ready to clean their microtome, the first thing to be done is to lock the hand wheel. Secondly, the disposable knife blade must be removed from the knife holder, and disposed of.
- Obviously, surgical grossing personnel must be aware of handling sharp blades as well, and exercise extreme caution.

Cuts should be treated with first aid immediately. The cut should have pressure applied to stop bleeding, and then be rinsed/soaked in Betadine before applying more pressure and a dressing. The patient should then be transported to the emergency room as soon as possible for treatment.

Waste streams

One of the best ways to ensure safety of laboratory employees from hazards is to mandate designated waste streams in the laboratory. The following are suggested.

- Biohazard waste
- Chemical waste
- Sharps waste
- Regular, sterile waste

Biohazard waste must be disposed of according to the Bloodborne Pathogens regulations. Specifically, biohazard waste must be double red-bagged before being placed into the final container for transport.

Sharps waste may ultimately go into the biohazard waste, if contaminated (i.e. surgical grossing blades, microtome blades). However, the blades, and any other sharps in the laboratory must be discarded into a red, hard plastic container first.

Chemical waste must first be segregated into the proper chemical waste streams (Figure 8). Your licensed waste chemical vendor will help you to determine the profile of each waste, such that it is stored and handled correctly, as well as being labelled correctly.

The remainder of laboratory waste is regular, sterile waste, generated in the lab. Paper towels used in handwashing, etc. fall into this category. Under no circumstances should any of the other three waste streams be discarded into the regular sterile waste stream. Following the above information and guidelines will help you to prevent injuries to you, your coworkers, and any other support staff that may enter and work in your laboratory.

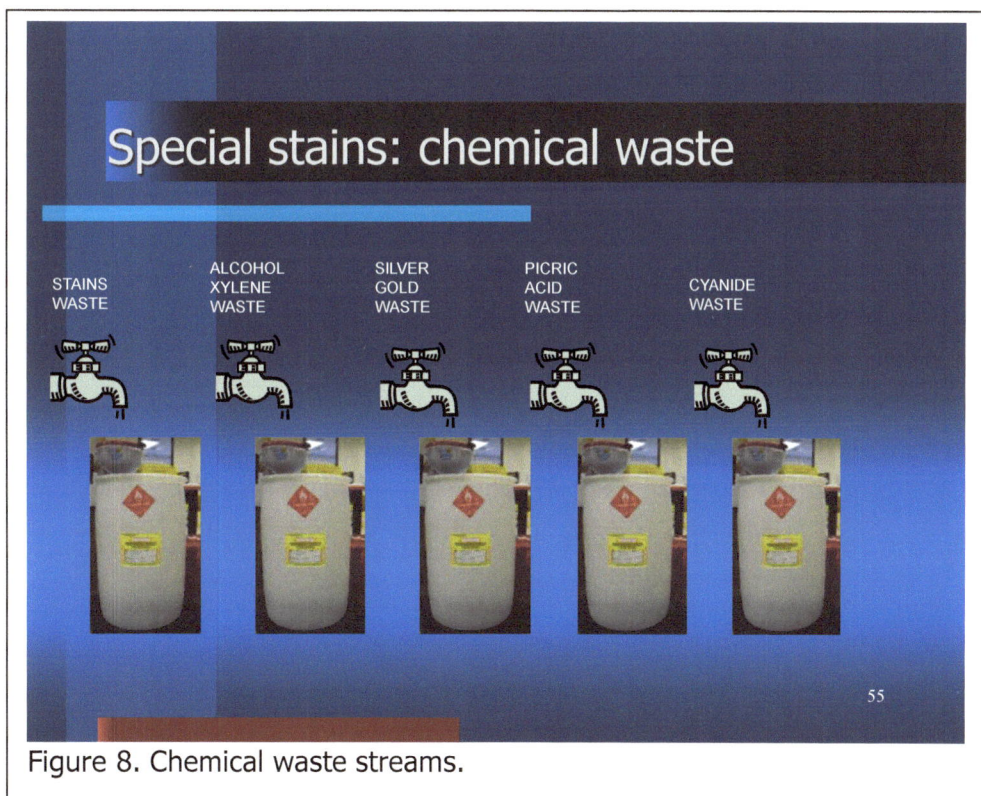

Figure 8. Chemical waste streams.

Handling Hazardous Waste

The US Environmental Protection Agency (EPA) defines waste as any solid, liquid or contained gas that is no longer used and is designated for disposal or recycling. If the waste can cause injury or death, or pollute land, water or air, it is deemed to be hazardous. EPA regulates hazardous waste at the federal level, and state regulation must be at least as stringent as the EPA.

In 1976, the Resource Conservation and Recovery Act (RCRA) were passed to track hazardous chemicals "from the cradle to the grave". RCRA defines two categories of hazardous waste:
- Listed waste is any substance appearing on any one of RCRA's four lists.
- Characteristic waste is any substance having one or more of the following characteristics:
    - Ignitability. This includes liquids with a flash point of less than 140 F (i.e. nearly all clearing agents and dehydrants/alcohols).
    - Corrosivity. This includes liquids with a pH less than or equal to 2.0, or greater than or equal to 12.5.
    - Reactivity. Substances that are unstable or undergo violent chemical reaction with water or other materials (i.e. picric acid).
    - TCLP toxicity. Substances that can leach from a secure landfill.

Strategies for Waste Handling

Recycling
Recycling makes the most sense. Alcohols, xylenes, xylene substitutes and formalin are examples of chemicals found in the histology laboratory that can be recycled. The laboratory is able to keep smaller quantities on site and recycling is very cost effective. Most recycling units pay for themselves in approximately two years.

Scaling Down
Make an attempt to "scale down" the quantities of chemicals that you use. For example, if you are performing an iron stain on two slides (i.e. patient and control) instead of using 50 ml in a Coplin jar, use 10 ml in a plastic slide holder. This decreases the amount of hazardous chemical waste you generate for this stain by more than half.

Re-use or "treat and release"

Non-mercury Harris' hematoxylin is an excellent candidate to be re-constituted and re-used after the first use. Then, once it is depleted, hematoxylin can be treated for drain disposal (with permission from the owner of your sanitary sewer).

Store for legal transport and disposal

This is the method of last resort. Alcohol tainted with xylene and special stains wastes fall into this category. These chemicals should be stored safely in drums for legal pick up and disposal by a licensed facility. Remember, even after the facility comes to pick up your waste – you still own it. If the waste hauler flips his truck over on the interstate, and your waste is on board – your laboratory helps pay for the clean up. If you are found negligent in handling your hazardous waste, there can be criminal charges, and you – yes you – can go to jail.

Substituting for Hazardous Chemicals

One strategy for decreasing the laboratory use of hazardous chemicals is to find substitutes for them. Ideally, a "safe" substitute is the best alternative. However, a "less hazardous" chemical also can help in this regard.

Fixation. Formaldehyde (i.e. formalin) has been the fixative of choice in histology laboratories for many years. However, you can see from the Formaldehyde Standard that many parameters must be met to insure employee safety when handling formalin. Spent formalin is considered to be a hazardous waste; however, it can be recycled.

Today, many formalin substitutes are available for fixation of tissue. One must be aware, however, that many of these substitutes are alcohol based. Formalin is a cross-linking fixative. Alcohol fixes tissue by denaturation. It is important to work with your pathologist to validate any changes in processing chemicals that are made, to ensure that the final slide is acceptable.

Dehydration. Dehydration of tissues during processing is still carried out by a graded alcohol series. Laboratories usually employ ethanol for this procedure.

Clearing. Xylene has been the clearing agent employed by laboratories for many years. It is similar to formalin in that proper ventilation must be used when handling it. Xylene is also easy to recycle.

Also like formalin, there are many xylene-substitutes available for use. Some are limonene based (i.e. citrus based). These are considered safe, however there are some reports indicating that some personnel may be allergic to them. Additionally, there are xylene-substitutes that are short-chain and long-chain aliphatic hydrocarbons. Whatever substitute is chosen, the laboratory should make certain to perform validations to insure specimen integrity. Additionally, all xylene substitutes can be recycled.

The most important aspect of using xylene substitutes (whether in processing or staining) is that they all are very water intolerant. Xylene can dissolve up to 3% water with no deleterious effect on processing or staining. Tissues and slides must be completely dehydrated prior to the xylene-substitute stations on the tissue processor and stainer to insure optimum quality. This requires a strict regimen of changing and rotating the 100% alcohols that precede the clearing step.

Incorporating some of these ideas may be time consuming. However, they will make your laboratory a safer place to work.

Chemistry 101

OK. I know that almost everyone hated taking chemistry in school.

However, in order to be a competent histologist that has the ability to troubleshoot processing and staining issues in the histology laboratory, you must have a basic understanding of how atoms and molecules bind together and react.

Atoms are the smallest building blocks of molecules. Atoms are composed of a nucleus, which contains protons and neutrons, that are surrounded by electrons. Protons have a positive charge, electrons have a negative charge, and neutrons are neutral – they have zero charge. One of the basic rules in chemistry is: opposites attract. This rule is the basis for atoms staying together: the negative electrons are attracted to the positive protons located inside the nucleus.

Back when I was in school (when the world was considered to be flat), atomic structure was likened to the planets orbiting the son: the nucleus was the sun, and the electrons orbited around it. Today, the facts support the idea of an "electron cloud" around each nucleus. Atoms may "share" their electron cloud with the same, or other different atoms, which binds them into molecules.

Figure 9 and 10 show how two separate hydrogen atoms bind together to make a hydrogen molecule. Hydrogen atoms are very stable when sharing their one electron, and this principle extends to all atoms: they "like" their first binding level of to be filled with two electrons. A carbon atom has a second, outer level that wants to be filled with eight electrons. It has four, so is always "looking" for four other atoms to share electrons with (Figure 11).

Histology involves using formaldehyde to chemically "fix" dynamic, living tissue into a static "snapshot" of cellular activity. The cells in your body are currently metabolizing energy sources, and performing chemical reactions to ensure that all of your bodily functions continue, and you stay alive. When tissue is removed from the body (i.e. surgery or biopsy), the cells no longer receive oxygen from the blood, and the cells begin to die, and autolyze (i.e. break down). The fixation process "fixes" the tissue, and stops the autolysis process, thereby preserving the cellular structure and tissue architecture, for subsequent processing into a paraffin block.

At the molecular level, formaldehyde is a simple molecule, consisting of one carbon atom joined to two hydrogen atoms with a single bond, and one oxygen atom with a double bond (Figure 12). Carbon is stable when it forms a total of four bonds. A double bond contains a lot of energy – similar to compressing a spring. The bond wants to "spring apart" to release the energy. It does this by "springing apart' the double bond, to provide two single bonds, which immediately bind two other molecules. This is what is meant by the term "cross linking" fixation, as relates to formaldehyde. The formaldehyde molecule cross links molecules within the protein structure of the cells (Figure 13).

Why do we need to know this?

Because living tissues are made up primarily of carbon, hydrogen and oxygen, and these are the molecules of biochemistry. Histologists need to know the chemistry of fixation, processing and staining.

Once the tissue is fixed in formalin, the proteins within are cross linked and stabilized. The tissue is in a solution of 4% formaldehyde in 96% water – similar to the natural water content of the human body. In routine histology, the final goal is to embed the tissue in a paraffin wax block. Water and wax do not mix. In order to be able to infiltrate the tissue with wax, and embed it in a paraffin block, the water has to be removed; the tissue must be dehydrated.

Dehydration is usually accomplished by using a graded series of alcohols to remove the water, and replace with 100% alcohol. Alcohol and wax do not mix. Therefore, histologists can use an "intermediate substance", to bridge the gap between alcohol and wax. For most laboratories, this substance is xylene – although there are now substitutes that can be used.

The molecular structure of xylene is shown in Figure 14. You can see that it is a "hybrid" molecule. The center is a "ring' of carbon atoms, with alternating single and double bonds. The exterior is made up of single bonds to hydrogen. This unique structure allows xylene to mix with both alcohol and paraffin. This brings us to the second rule of chemistry: "like dissolves like". The middle ring of xylene is described as "organic", which is like the organic ring structure of paraffin. The exterior is a straight chain "inorganic" structure, which is like the structure of alcohol.

The principles above form the basis of understanding the chemical basis of fixation and processing of tissues in histology. Once you understand them, you can troubleshoot fixation and processing issues that will occur in your laboratory.

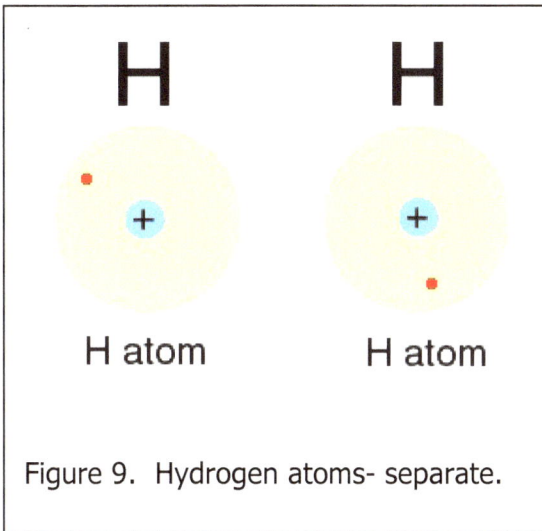

Figure 9. Hydrogen atoms- separate.

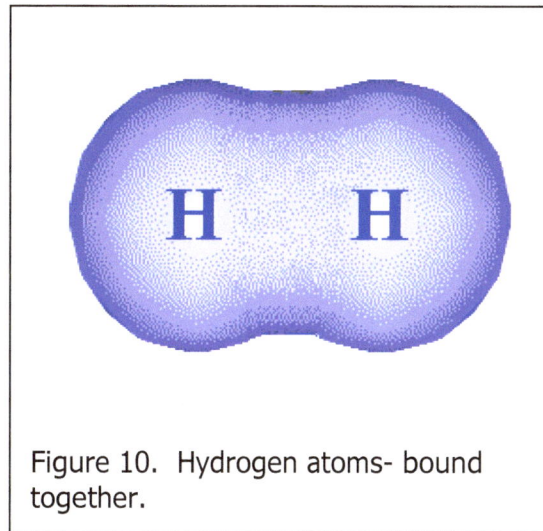

Figure 10. Hydrogen atoms- bound together.

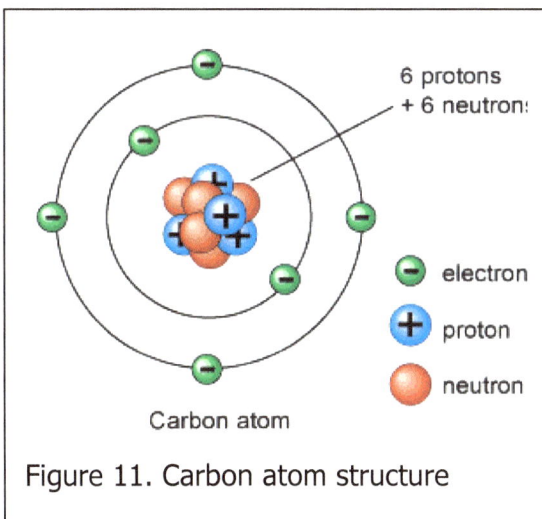

6 protons + 6 neutrons

− electron

+ proton

neutron

Carbon atom

Figure 11. Carbon atom structure

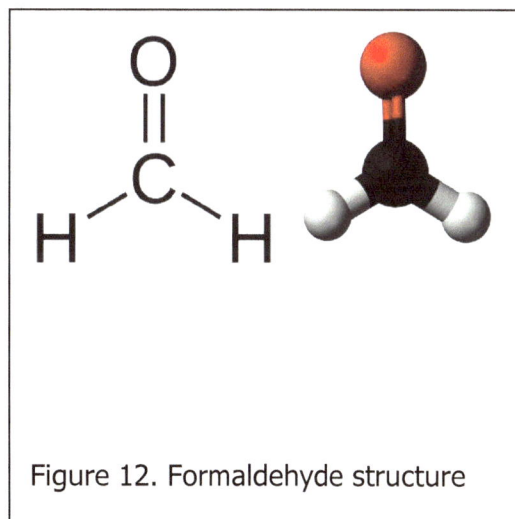

Figure 12. Formaldehyde structure

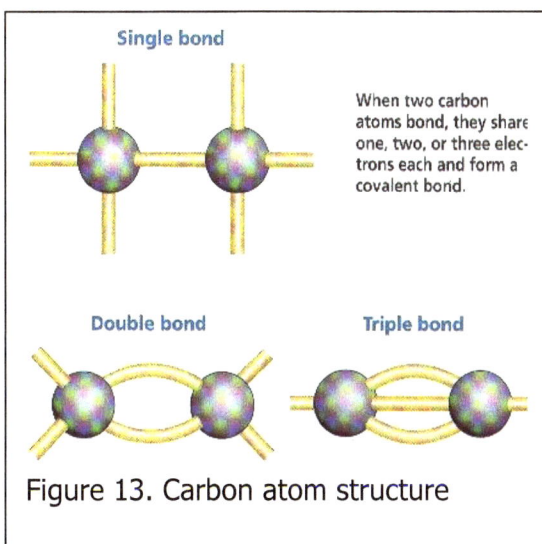

Single bond

When two carbon atoms bond, they share one, two, or three electrons each and form a covalent bond.

Double bond   **Triple bond**

Figure 13. Carbon atom structure

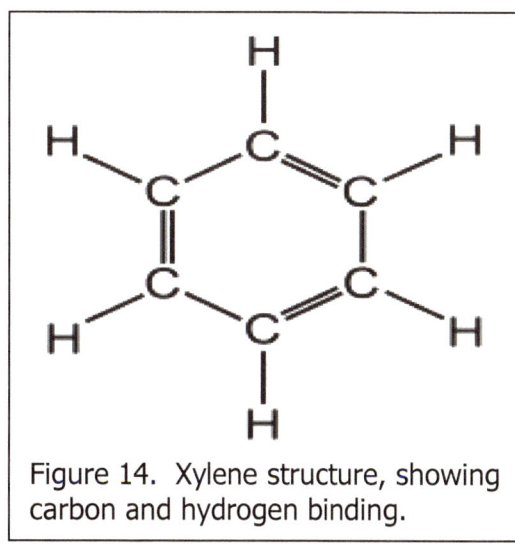

Figure 14. Xylene structure, showing carbon and hydrogen binding.

29

Chemistry 102

OK. I know the previous Chemistry 101 may have traumatized you a bit. But hang in there – we're almost done.

The dyes used in histology are chemical dyes that react in accordance with the basic rules of chemistry. Whether you are performing a routine hematoxylin and eosin (H&E) stain, or a special stain for fungi, the staining methods are based on underlying chemical principles.

The most basic chemical principle is that of pH, which is a figure expressing the acidity or alkalinity of a solution on a logarithmic scale on which 7 is neutral, lower values are more acid, and higher values more alkaline. The "p" stands for potential and the "H" stands for hydrogen. pH is the negative log of hydrogen ion concentration in a water-based solution. Figure 15 shows the pH scale, with some examples of acidic and basic solutions. Acidic solutions have extra "H + " molecules, and basic solutions have extra "OH - " molecules. Remember from Chemistry 101? Rule #1 in chemistry is: opposites attract.

Basic and Acidic Dyes
The most widely used histological stains differentiate between the acidic and basic components of cells and tissues. Acids and bases are defined by the measure of their pH. Basic dyes have a net positive charge. They bind to components of cells and tissues that are negatively charged. Examples include: hematoxylin, phosphate groups of nucleic acids (DNA and RNA), sulfate groups of some polysaccharides (glycosaminoglycans) and some proteins (mucus). Tissue components that stain with basic dyes are referred to as basophilic.

Acidic dyes have a net negative charge. They bind to components of cells and tissues that are positively charged. Examples include: eosin and ionized amino groups in proteins (side chains of lysine and arginine). Tissue components that stain with acid dyes are referred to as acidophilic.

The first use of a dye is credited to Antonie van Leeuwenhoek who, in 1673, worked with "saffron", a natural dye extracted from saffron crocus to stain histological structures, but genuine work on histological dye staining started not before the second half of the 19th century when C Weigher, J Gerlach, P Erlich and H Gierke systematically studied dyes for histology. At that time coloring materials were still of natural origin from which carmine or cochineal was the most used dye.

The human eye is able to perceive wavelengths of light between 400 and 700 nm. Dyes appear colored because they absorb a particular wavelength in the visible region, and the eye senses the reflected light as the complementary color.

According to their sources, coloring agents are discerned as natural or as synthetic dyes. So-called general stains will dye the tissue uniformly (indifferently) while selective stains have affinity for special cell or tissue components. A new chapter in the history of staining began when WH Perkin discovered the first aniline dye (from extracts of coal tar) in 1856 which would revolutionize the dying industry.

Dyes can be roughly divided into acidic dyes and basic dyes. Basic dyes stain acidic components, and acidic dyes stain mainly basic components. Histological staining is usually done by staining of cut sections inasmuch as a dye in solution is offered to bind to defined tissue structures. Progressive and regressive techniques can be differentiated including direct and indirect procedures.

One can operate with mixtures of dyes simultaneously or successively in order to discriminate different tissue textures by the respective dyes used. So, double, triple and multiple staining can be achieved. Many dyes have only poor affinity to tissues, but this can be overcome by the use of metal salts. Those enhancing compounds are then called "mordants". A uniform theory of histological dye staining does not exist. This is because the mechanisms of dye binding to the different tissue components are quite heterogeneous.

The Chemistry of Hematoxylin & Eosin (H&E)

Hematoxylin and eosin, H&E or HE stain is the most commonly used technique in histology. This stain works well with a variety of fixatives and displays a broad range of cytoplasmic, nuclear, and extracellular matrix features.

Hematoxylin is a positively charged, blue dye complex. It stains basophilic structures, such as nuclei. Eosin is a negatively charged, pink dye. It stains acidophilic (also known as eosinophilic) structures. Some structures do not stain well with H&E. Hydrophobic structures tend to remain clear (such as those rich in fats).

The hallmark of an excellent H&E stain is the presence of all nuclei stained with precise differentiation, showing chromatin material, and nucleoli. In addition, the eosin stain should result in three shades of pink: (1) bright pink red blood cells, (2) medium pink staining of compact connective tissue and (3) light pink staining of loose connective tissue. Figure16 shows such an H&E stain.

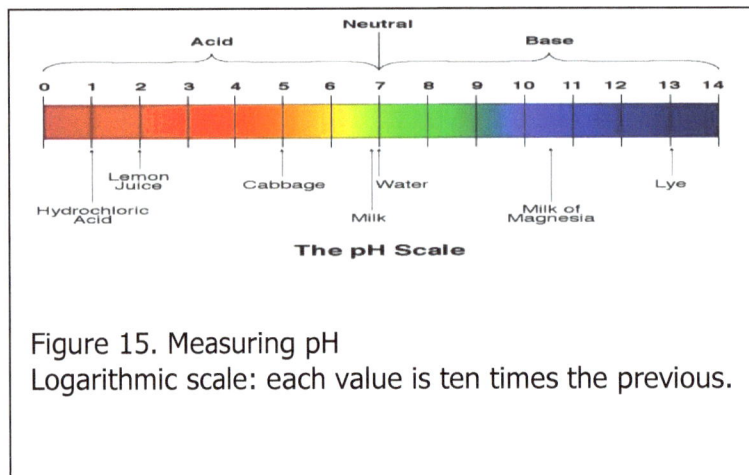

Figure 15. Measuring pH
Logarithmic scale: each value is ten times the previous.

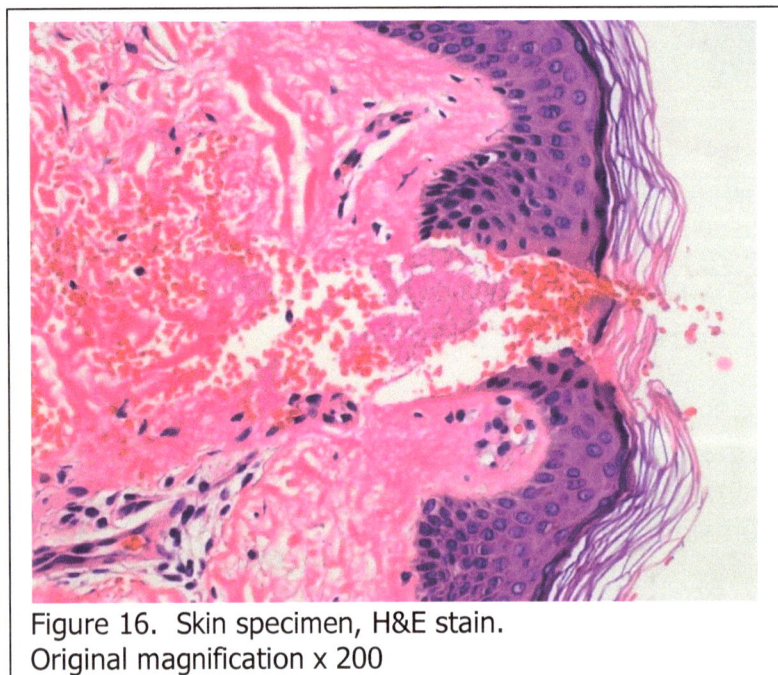

Figure 16. Skin specimen, H&E stain.
Original magnification x 200

Proper receipt of specimens

If you have worked in the histology field for some time, as I have, you may have noticed that the specimens you receive in your laboratory are getting smaller. This is not due to our failing eyesight. Instead, the advances in immunohistochemistry (IHC) and molecular techniques now enable the pathologist to make diagnoses on smaller and smaller fragments of tissue obtained during biopsy procedures. This fact, along with the emphasis on greater patient care quality, requires that each and every specimen received in your laboratory must be routed to the correct area, and handled appropriately.

In non-specialty hospital and private reference histology laboratories, the vast majority of specimens are received in 10% neutral buffered formalin for "routine histology". This means specimens will undergo surgical grossing procedures and routine processing through graded alcohols, xylene and paraffin embedding. Initial hematoxylin and eosin (H&E) stained slides will be prepared from paraffin blocks. Upon review by a pathologist, a diagnosis is rendered. Some cases may require additional IHC, molecular and/or special stains to confirm the diagnosis.

Some specimens may be received in formalin into the routine lab; however, they may require "non-routine" handling. Skin specimens submitted for "Slow Mohs" processing are such specimens. These are pieces of skin that are carefully marked with colored inks to indicate exact orientation. Laboratory personnel who receive the specimens, and who perform the surgical grossing techniques must recognize these "up front". Failure to recognize such specimens may result in changing/destroying the orientation, resulting in the pathologist's inability to render an accurate diagnosis with regard to tumor location with respect to surgical margins.

Similarly, a two millimeter punch specimen of skin may be mishandled by laboratory staff, if not identified "up front" at the time of receipt. These specimens should be identified for embedding and microtomy personnel. The microtomy personnel must pick up the very first sections, and observe the unstained slide under the microscope to ensure correct dermal-epidermal orientation Figures 17,18). If the specimen has been mis-embedded, there is enough tissue to melt down and re-embed correctly. Failure to follow this procedure may result in the production of initial and level slides that are mis-embedded. The final result may be that the specimen cannot be diagnosed.

An inherent danger exists in the minority of specimens that may be received for unique, specialized procedures. If these specimens are received in the incorrect fixative, or routed into the "routine histology" workflow, they may be unable to be used in the specialized procedures for which they were sent to the laboratory.

Specimens for direct immunofluorescence (DIF) are usually skin and kidney biopsies. Clinicians must be educated <u>to ensure that these specimens are not fixed in formalin.</u> Instead, these specimens must be submitted in "Michel's transport medium", sometimes labelled "Immuno transport fluid". This solution contains ammonium sulfate, which acts to precipitate proteins at their precise site of localization. This enables the frozen sections prepared to be stained with fluorescein labelled antibody preparations, in order to pinpoint the exact histological location of the proteins in question. Use of formalin fixation causes crosslinking of these proteins, which subsequently changes the antigenicity, making the proteins unable to be recognized by the antibodies.

Two specimen types may be received for urate crystal evaluation: both tissues and fluids may be submitted by clinicians. Joint fluids obtained by fine needle aspiration may be submitted – still contained within the syringe. <u>These specimens must not be fixed in formalin or cytology fixatives.</u> Instead, the fluid should be dispensed on to a clean, labelled microscope slide, using ventilation and Universal Precautions (i.e. the fluid may contain active, blood borne pathogens). After air drying, the slide is cover slipped with Permount and observed under polarizing light.

Similarly, a tissue specimen must be submitted in either Carnoy's fixative (chloroform and absolute ethanol) or simply absolute ethanol. Fixation cannot be in formalin, as formalin contains water which may dissolve any urate crystals that are present. Once received, the specimen must be processed from 100% ethanol, skipping over the formalin and graded alcohol series in the tissue processor. Once processing and embedding are complete, a slide for H&E and an unstained slide should be prepared. The unstained slide should be rinsed in xylene to remove the paraffin, and then cover slipped. As described above, the unstained slide is viewed under polarized light. Urate crystals will appear as bright white needles on a black background (Figures 19, 20).

In summary, it is excellent practice to identify any and all specimens that may be received by your laboratory for "non-routine" histology. Once identified, procedures should be developed for proper receipt and handling of the specimens. This is the only way to ensure the highest patient care quality.

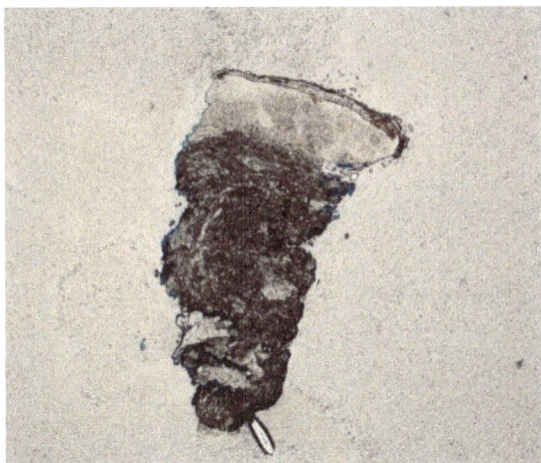

Figure 17.
Skin, 2 mm punch specimen
Unstained
Original magnification x10

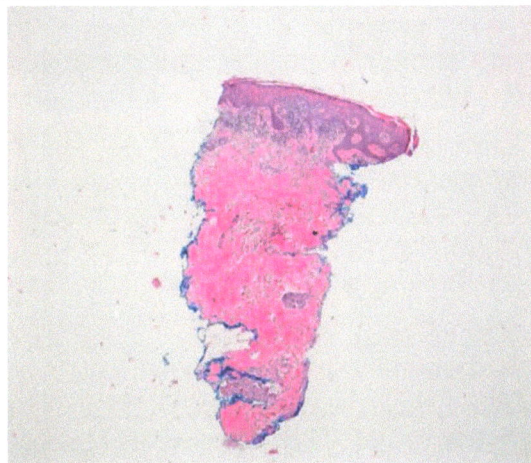

Figure 18.
Skin, 2 mm punch specimen
H&E
Original magnification x10

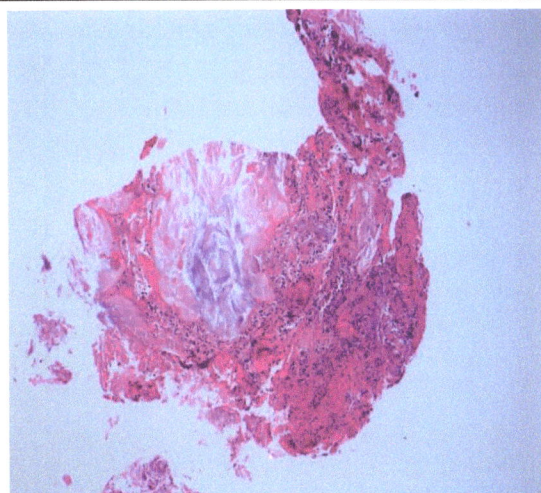

Figure 19.
Skin, H&E
Gout preparation
Original magnification x40

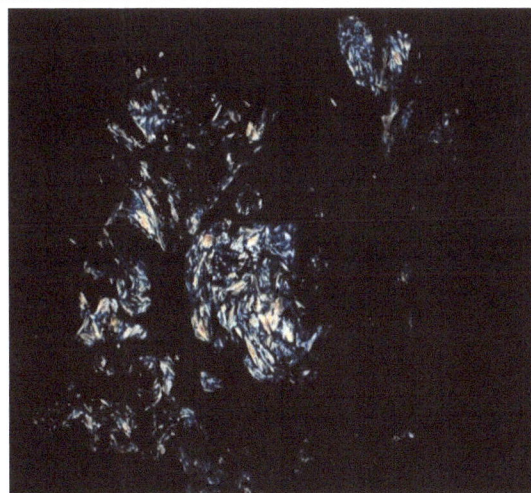

Figure 20. Skin, polarized light
Gout preparation
Original magnification x40

Surgical Grossing: Special Cases

There are some unique specimens received in the histology laboratory that may cause problems for the histologist if not handled properly at the time of surgical grossing. The following specimen types are described and specific procedures are recommended for their successful handling in the *Procedures* section of the laboratory manual "Dermatopathology Laboratory Techniques" by Clifford M. Chapman and Dr. Izak Dimenstein (2016).

Skin specimens for alopecia
   Skin specimens may be taken from the scalp in order to determine if the patient is suffering from alopecia (hair loss).   These are almost always punch specimens, and are usually 3-4 mm in diameter. In order to count hair follicles for comparison, these are the only skin specimens that are not cut perpendicular to the dermal-epidermal junction. Rather, they are cut parallel to it, resulting in cross sections of the hair follicles. This method was developed by Dr. Headington, and is referred to as the Headington procedure.

Skin specimens for Direct Immunofluorescence (DIF)
   Skin specimens may be taken from lesional, sun exposed and non-sun exposed areas from patients by dermatologists who suspect the patients may have bullous (blistering) or autoimmune (i.e. lupus) diseases. In these cases, two specimens are usually submitted: one in formaldehyde, the other in Immunofluorescence Transport Medium. This medium may also be referred to as Michel's medium, named after the doctor who developed it. The medium consists of buffered ammonium sulfate that acts to fix proteins at their site within the skin specimen. Once received in the laboratory, the specimens are washed in buffer and frozen in cryostat embedding medium for cryostat sectioning and subsequent staining with immunofluorescence reagents. It is imperative that specimens submitted for DIF not be fixed in formaldehyde. Once a specimen is exposed to formaldehyde, it is rendered useless for DIF.

Tiny specimens
Some specimens may be very tiny; on the order of less than 0.1 cm. Some methods employ the use of mesh cassettes, "tea bag" biopsy pouches, sponges, wrapping paper, etc. in order to contain the specimen and prevent it from escaping the tissue processing cassette. A disadvantage of the above methods is that upon embedding, the specimen has to be handled yet again, possibly resulting in additional fragmentation of the tissue, or possibly complete tissue loss.

A proper method of using wrapping papers is described by Dr. Izak B Dimenstein in his Technical Note published in the Journal of Histotechnology (2016. Vol. 39, No. 3, pages 76-80). This method works very well for fragile tissues such as prostate and breast needle biopsies. Dr. Dimenstein notes that use of sponges/polyester pads may result in a 'compression artefact", which can occur during processing. Specifically, tissue needle biopsies may compress and narrow, comparable to the size of the pad mesh holes. One solution is to lay out and wrap the core in lens paper, and then sandwich the wrapped specimen between two sponges, which have been pre-soaked in formalin.

With regard to core fragments remaining in the specimen bottle, Dr. Dimenstein recommends filtration through a porous paper, such as the internal layer of a Kimberly-Clark protective mask. This is more reliable than trying to remove fragments with a pipette, where mucous or tiny fragments may stick to the inside of the pipette. He does not recommend filtration through nylon mesh bags, as the tiny fragments are difficult to retrieve during embedding.

With regard to embedding, Dr. Dimenstein recommends the use of a tamper to flatten the core, to keep it parallel to the block face. If two cores are present, they should be embedded parallel to each other, and to the horizontal axis of the block. Filtration specimens should be embedded in the manner similar to embedding any aggregate of tissue, carefully grouping the fragments into the middle of the mold.

In addition to the above method, Sakura Finetek has a product called "embedding gel" that can be used in conjunction with their Paraform cassettes. This material can be used to hold small specimens in place, in proper orientation.

An alternative method is to use a product called "HistoGel". HistoGel is a liquid at 55 C, and has a gelatin consistency at room temperature. The idea is simply to surround the tiny tissue fragment(s) with liquefied HistoGel, allow it to cool to room temperature (two minutes), thereby trapping the tissue fragment in the HistoGel, much the same way fruit is embedded in the gelatin of a Jell-O fruit mold. The resulting "button" of HistoGel containing the tissue is placed into a tissue processing cassette and processed as usual. (Note: do not use microwave processing, or "Rush" processing.) During embedding, the button is simply removed from the cassette and embedded as usual. Additional slides may have to be taken in order to reach the fragment; however, *the tissue cannot be lost in processing*. This fact far outweighs the extra effort involved during the surgical grossing procedure.

Figure 21A shows a black ink dot, marking the presence of a small group of cells that represent a tiny fragment submitted in HistoGel. Figure 21B is a high power micrograph of the specimen stained with PAS. Fungi are clearly demonstrated. The specimen was so small that it had to be serially sectioned. Slides #5, 6, and 7 out of 30 slides showed the tissue fragment.

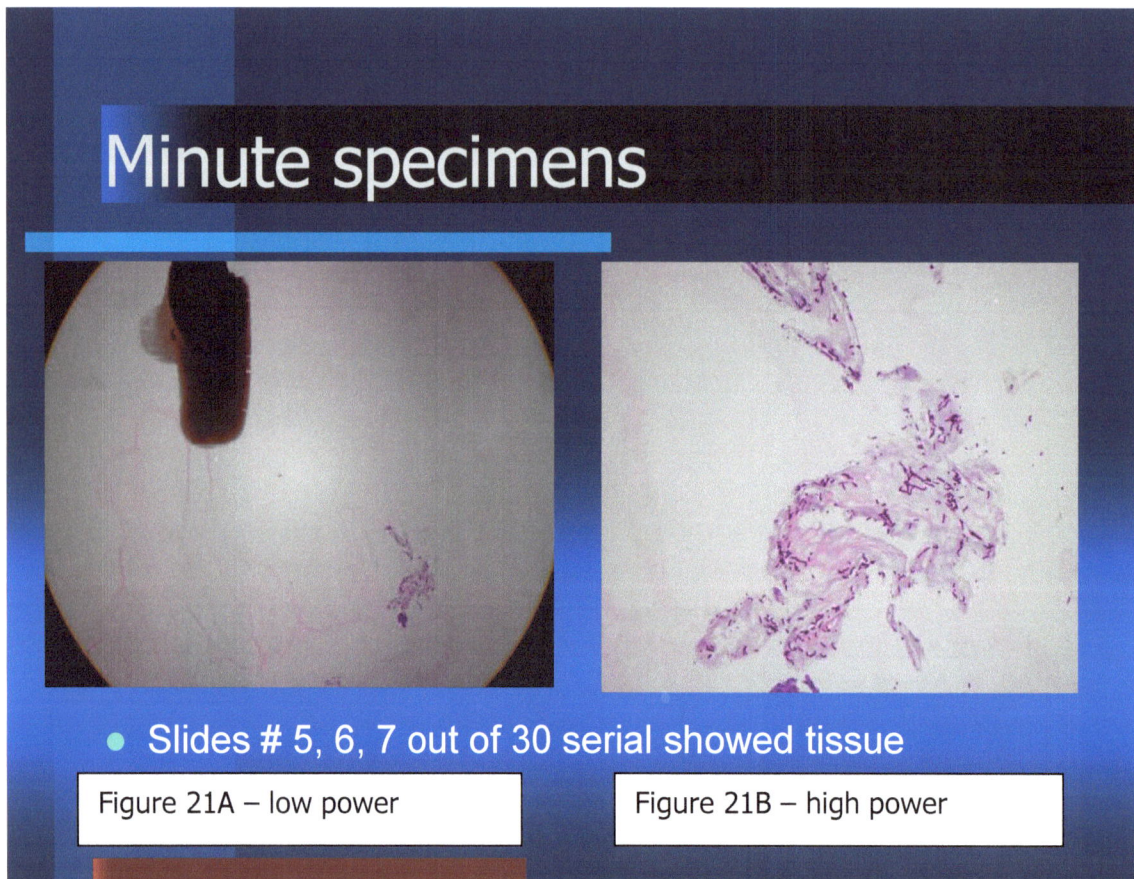

Minute specimens

- Slides # 5, 6, 7 out of 30 serial showed tissue

Figure 21A – low power

Figure 21B – high power

Nail specimens

Fingernail or toenail specimens may be received in the laboratory for histology. Usually, the clinician suspects a fungal infection, however, in some cases, a malignant melanoma may be suspected. In either case, the nail must first be fixed thoroughly in formaldehyde. After fixation, the nail should be held overnight in nail softening solution, which will soften and continue to fix the nail. The following day, the specimen may be processed routinely into a paraffin block. After cutting, the sections should be picked up on gelatin coated slides. This insures that the sections will adhere to the slide during H&E, PAS and immunohistochemical staining.

Bone specimens

How can one tissue behave like Dr. Jekyll and the other like Mr. Hyde? As with many things in histology, the answer is in the details. The histologist must understand the histology of bone tissue in order to produce optimal microscope slides.

Everyone knows that bone is basically hard and brittle. This characteristic is due to the cell biology of bone growth and development. Bone collagen is laid down in bands that are parallel to one another. These bands, or lamellae, become mineralized with a polysaccharide containing calcium and phosphate which provides strength necessary in cortical bone to provide support to the skeleton. Trabecular bone is mineralized in a similar fashion, however, many spaces remain where bone marrow is located. The bone marrow stem cells divide and grow into the specialized blood cell components (Figure 22).

Bone is a dynamic, living tissue. New bone is made by osteoblasts located on the surface of newly formed bone. The most recent material is not mineralized and is referred to as the osteoid seam. This material is mineralized later to form mature bone. Osteoclasts are also located on the bone surface. These are large, multinucleated cells responsible for "eating up" mature bone to release calcium into the blood stream. If the balance between these two bone cell types is disturbed, disease may result. Osteoporosis is a disease where the osteoclast activity outpaces the osteoblast activity; weak, porotic bones prone to breakage, can result (Figure 23).

The million dollar question in the histology laboratory is: How can we prepare bone specimens to be cut from a paraffin block on a rotary microtome, and keep the sections on the slide for optimal staining?

As with all specimens, the answer begins with proper fixation. The "20 to 1" rule applies in that the bone specimen should be placed into unbuffered formalin fixative, in a volume that is 20 times that of the size of the specimen. Then, since bone is very dense, the fixation time should be measured in days – not hours; with an average of 3-5 days of fixation for larger specimens.

Once the specimen is fixed, it must be decalcified. Methods must be used that will remove the calcium from the bone tissue, to render it soft and amenable to subsequent processing and cutting. There are methods for processing mineralized bone into plastic, however these methods are not within the scope of this discussion.

Before we discuss what can be used as decalcifying agents, we must understand that all act in the same way. That is, the solutions are used to leach out and remove calcium ions from the tissue. To that end, specimens should be placed into a decalcifying solution that is 100 times the volume of the specimen, thereby provided plenty of solution. Since the solution will now become saturated with calcium during the process, it should be changed every 24 hours. Large pieces of bone should be cut with a scalpel into smaller pieces as they become softer, yielding pieces of tissue not exceeding 2 mm in thickness. Finally, the solution should be agitated using a rotary shaker, or stirring mechanism (Figure 24).

So then, what decalcifying solution should be used? Below are a few that are currently in use:

Rapid decalcifer: These solutions usually contain hydrochloric and/or nitric acid, and are used on bone marrow biopsies. The advantage of rapid decalcifying over some hours is offset by decreased histology quality, and possibility of antigenicity damage.

Bouin's solution: The picric acid contained in Bouin's solution can decalcify bone in small bone marrow biopsies, as described above. The disadvantage is that picric acid is a dangerous chemical to use and dispose of.

10% formic acid in 10% unbuffered formaldehyde: This method yields the best histology. The disadvantage of this solution is the time it takes to decalcify is measured in days.

Chelating agents: These are mostly used in research applications, as histology and antigenicity are maximally preserved. However, the time frame is measured in weeks.

The endpoint of decalcification can be determined subjectively, via manual manipulation of the tissue to determine softness. Conversely, the chemical method detailed in the procedure "Determining the Endpoint of Decalcification", [Procedures Section] can be used (Luna, 1968). After decalcification is complete, the tissue should be rinsed thoroughly in running tap water. Processing should be done using a procedure for large, dense tissues.

During microtomy, if there are times that the decalcification seems to be incomplete, the histologist may soak the block face in decalcification solution for 30 minutes to an hour. Then, after rinsing, the first few sections should cut easier and be floated out on the water bath for section pick up. Finally, microscope slides coated with 0.5% gelatin should be used to pick up sections. This will help the sections to adhere to the microscope slide during staining. Some eosin background staining on the slide may result, but it does not affect the final H and E stain.

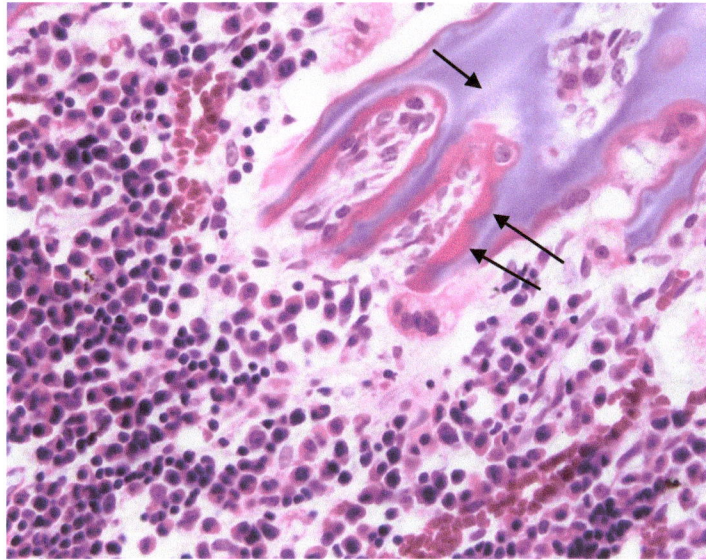

Figure 22. Decalcified bone section, HE stain showing lamellar bone (arrow) and osteoid seam (double arrow), with adjacent bone marrow.
Original magnification x 200

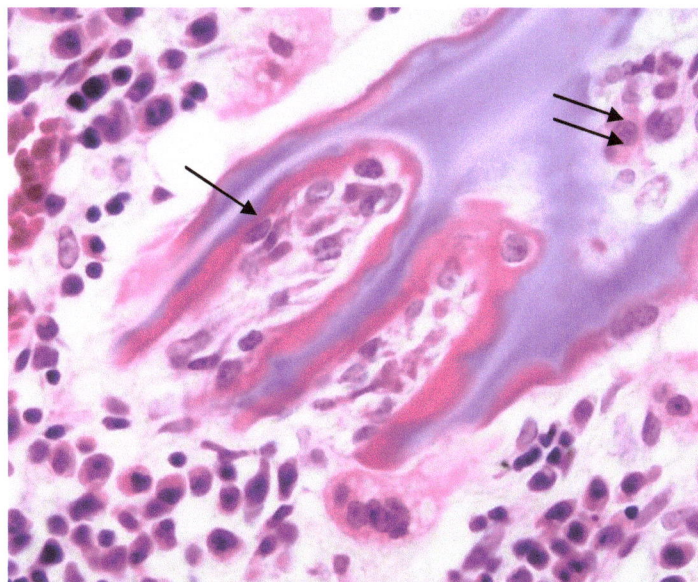

Figure 23. Osteoblast (arrow) and osteoclast (double arrow), HE stain.
Original magnification x 600

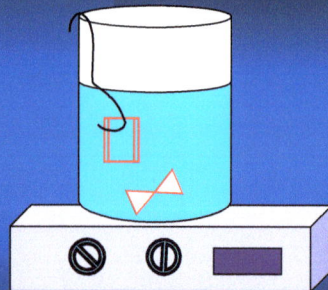

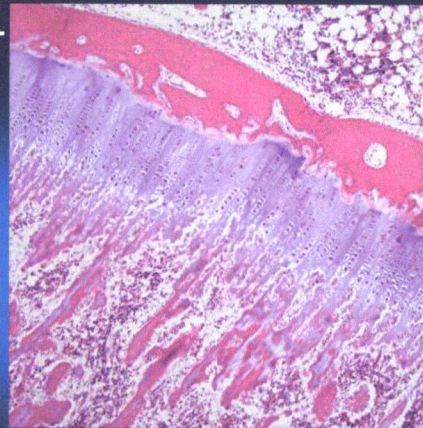

Figure 24. Suggested apparatus for decalcification of bone.

Skin Specimens and Dermatopathology

In order to successfully prepare slides of skin specimens, the histologist must understand basic skin histology. Two major reasons for this are:

- The pathologist must be able to see the dermal-epidermal junction. The vast majority of skin pathology takes place in this area.
- Skin specimens are composed of three major tissue areas: epidermis, dermis and sub-cutaneous (adipose). This has ramifications for processing and cutting.

Dermatopathology is a subject heading in pathology all unto itself. The intrinsic nature of dermatopathology specimens received in a laboratory necessitates a clear understanding of the material due to importance of the skin's histology presentation as an organ. The goal of the histologist in the preparation of dermatopathology slides is to ensure that the entire area of skin which may contain pathology is represented in the final microscope slide. A detailed discussion of dermatopathology is out of the realm of this publication. However, this information is readily available in the publication *Dermatopathology Laboratory Techniques* written by CM Chapman and IB Dimenstein which is available on line at Amazon.com.

Hair Specimens

There are instances when the histology laboratory will receive a hair specimen from a patient for diagnosis. This is not to be confused with residual hair left on a skin specimen. Sometimes, hair itself is obtained by pulling it from the scalp, in order to determine any pathology that might be present.

Hair specimens for genetic disorders are usually submitted unfixed. In these cases, the pathologist will require that the hairs simply be submitted on a microscope slide with a coverglass, held in place with a drop or two of mounting medium to keep the hair in place. The hair is then viewed by the pathologist, unstained, under light microscopy. An example of such a preparation is shown in Figures 25 and 26. Monilethrix is a disease that may also be referred to as "beaded hair". Patients present with short, fragile broken hair. This condition is caused by a genetic mutation for which there is no treatment.

More commonly, hair specimens may be submitted to the histology laboratory for diagnosis of trichomycosis, which is a general term for fungal infection of the hair.

There are some technical challenges presented when a hair specimen reaches the histology laboratory and requires a PAS stain for fungi (Figures 27, 28). The hair strands must be handled gently with forceps, as the surgical grossing is performed and the specimen described. The specimen should not be processed into a paraffin block

43

for routine H&E staining. Instead, the hairs should be transferred to a 20 ml glass scintillation vial (or similar container) in order for the PAS stain to be performed manually. The staining solutions are transferred by using a disposable 3 ml plastic bulb pipette. In this way, the hairs are retained in the container. Solutions should be discarded into a beaker, in order to prevent any of the hair strands from being lost [see Procedures Section].

Monilethrix

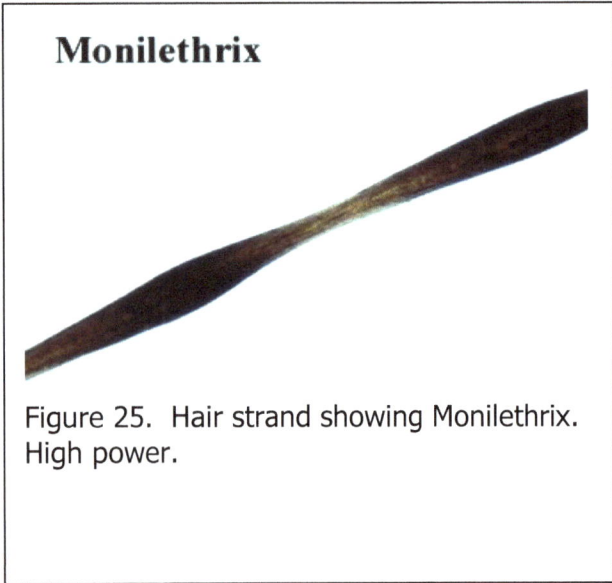

Figure 25. Hair strand showing Monilethrix. High power.

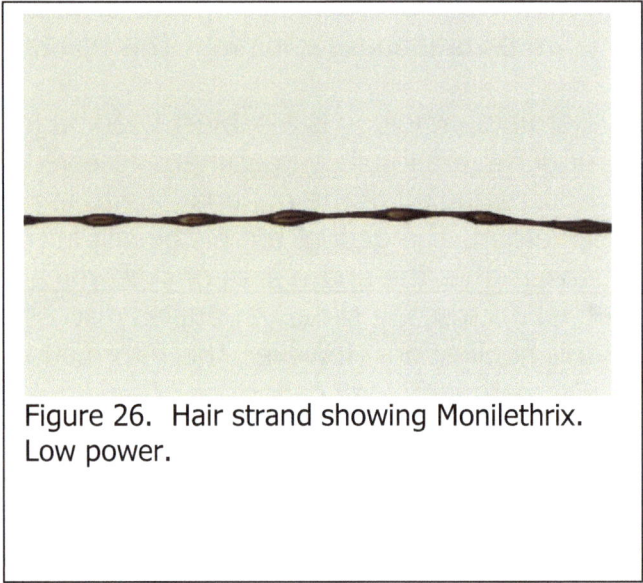

Figure 26. Hair strand showing Monilethrix. Low power.

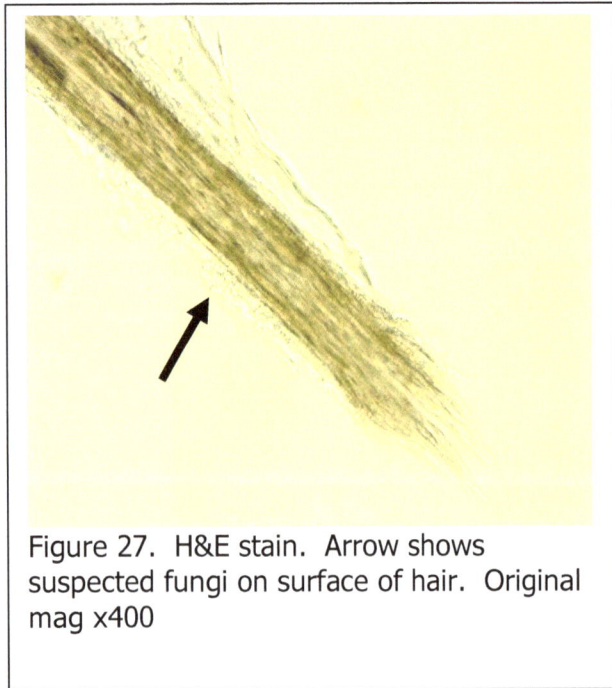

Figure 27. H&E stain. Arrow shows suspected fungi on surface of hair. Original mag x400

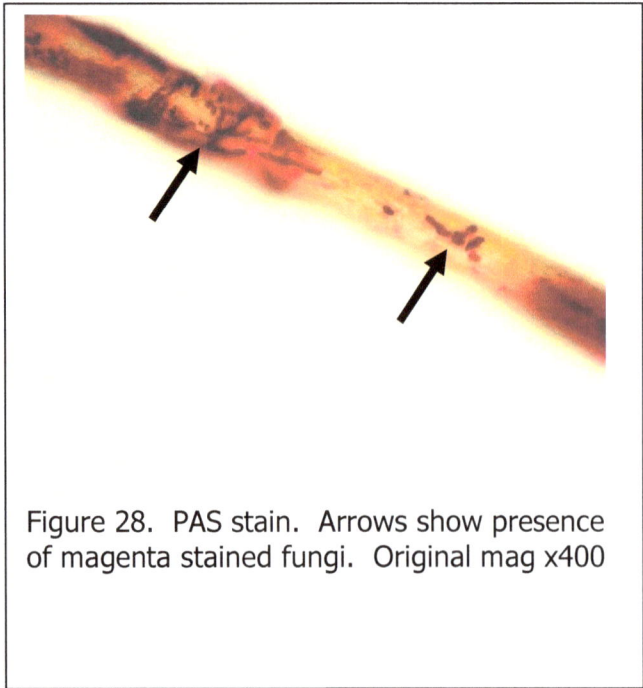

Figure 28. PAS stain. Arrows show presence of magenta stained fungi. Original mag x400

Prostate

Whether you work in a hospital laboratory or a private reference laboratory, you probably receive specimens of prostate gland. In a hospital setting, the specimen may be received from a transurethral resection of the prostate, or a surgical resection of the entire prostate gland. In both cases, large pieces of prostate tissue are submitted to the pathology laboratory. In a private reference laboratory, usually needle core biopsies of the prostate are received (see Figure 29). These specimens usually measure approximately 1 mm in diameter by 1 cm long (Figure 30). Multiple needle core biopsies are usually procured from different areas within the prostate.

The prostate gland is comprised of many glands, with associated ducts, surrounded by connective tissue (Figure 31). The pathologist must assess the glandular areas and determine if there are any cancer cells present. Sometimes the diagnosis can be made with a hematoxylin and eosin (H&E) stained slide (Figure 32). Other times, the H&E slide may not be conclusive (Figure 33). In this case, immunohistochemical (IHC) stains must be performed (Figure 34).

A multi- antibody IHC stain can be used on prostate sections to assist in demonstrating if cancer cells are present. A high molecular weight cytokeratin cocktail of clones CK5 and CK14 are used to stain basal epithelia in the prostate gland. The P504S protein is known to be expressed by prostate adenocarcinoma cells, but not in benign prostate cells. It may also be produced by high grade prostatic intraepithelial neoplasia (PIN). Finally, the p63 antibody is added to the cocktail to detect normal cells, and is not produced by malignant tumor cells. The results of the staining patterns are used to confirm or rule out prostate cancer and prostatic intraepithelial neoplasia (Figure 34).

Initial receipt and handling of prostate needle cores must be done with care. The cores are small, fragile and easily damaged. Many times they are received fragmented. The exact number of cores and fragments must be documented during the surgical grossing procedure. These specimens must be wrapped, or contained in some way to prevent escape from the tissue cassette. The Sakura ParaForm cassettes are an option in this regard.

Processing may be done using routine tissue processing through alcohols, xylene and paraffin. A short biopsy protocol should be used to prevent over-dehydration of the tissue. Alternatively, a microwave assisted processor may be used. The omission of xylene during this processing protocol ensures that needle cores remain soft for optimal microtomy.
The same care taken in surgical grossing must be utilized during the embedding procedure. Tissues must be unwrapped and handled gently to prevent fragmentation

of the cores. Also, the cores must be embedded completely flat, to ensure accurate representation of the tissue in the final microscope slide.

Great care must be taken by histologists when cutting prostate needle cores. Usually, multiple, shallow levels are taken and picked up on 5 separate slides. Slides 1, 3 and 5 are stained with H&E. Slides 2 and 4 are held, unstained, for use in the IHC staining with the PIN 4 cocktail. Preservation of tissue is of the utmost importance.

The resulting stained slides are able to be used to obtain the maximum amount of information regarding any pathology present in these tiny specimens. Pathologists are able to assess and grade the prostate cancer, if present. This information is relayed to the clinician to help determine the treatment and prognosis of the patient.

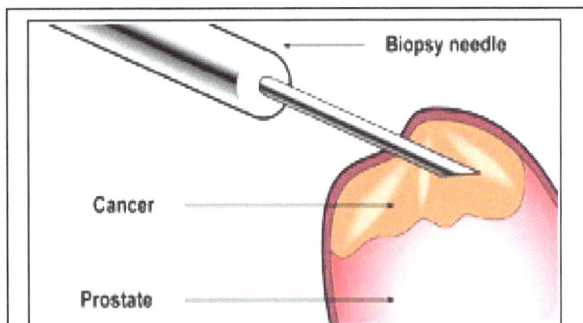

Figure 6: Needle Biopsy

Figure 29. Needle core biopsy of prostate gland.

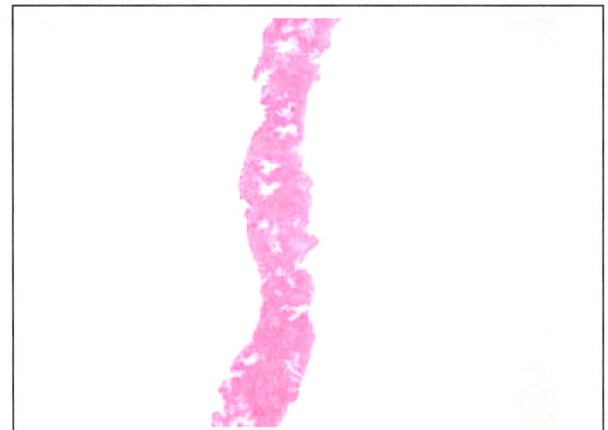

Figure 30. Prostate needle core biopsy stained with H&E.
Original magnification x2.

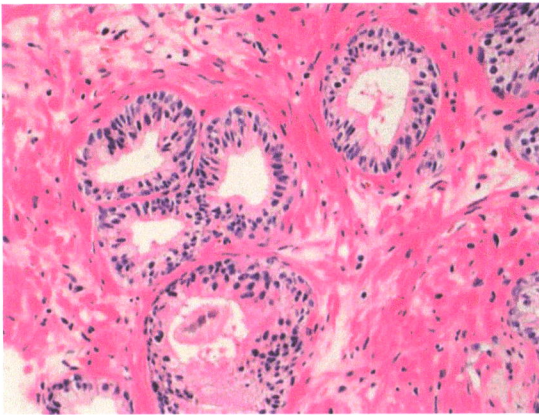

Figure 31. H&E stain of prostate gland within needle biopsy showing normal cells.
Original magnification x 40.

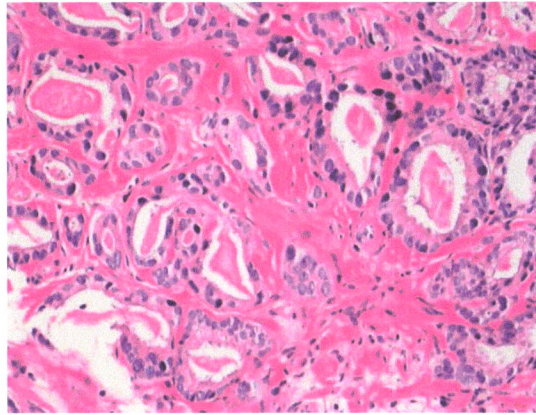

Figure 32. H&E stain of prostate gland within needle biopsy showing cancer cells.
Original magnification x 40.

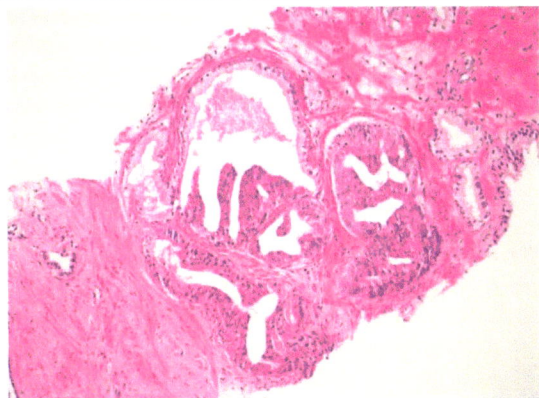

Figure 33. Prostate needle core biopsy stained with H&E showing glandular structure. Original magnification x20.

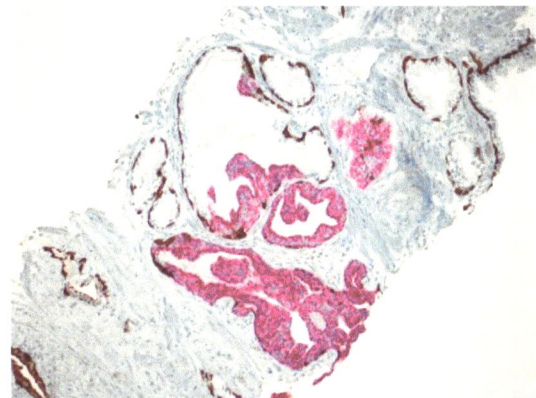

Figure 34. Serial section next to Figure 33, showing PIN 4 staining. Red chromogen stains P504S, while brown stains p63 and HMW cytokeratin. Original magnification x20.

Neuropathology

Neuropathology is a histology specialty unto itself. Most hospitals and healthcare facilities will refer patients to a neuropathology center. Specimens can be procured by neurosurgery (i.e. tumor samples, brain biopsies, peripheral nerve biopsies, skeletal muscle biopsy) or post mortem (i.e. whole brain or spinal cord).

While your laboratory may not receive neuropathology specimens, there may be times when you might be consulted regarding fixation and processing of such specimens. Brain and spinal cord biopsies are tiny in nature, and the specimens are usually "sticky". Parafilm or a piece of polythene, folded over to prevent drying, may be used to receive and transport fresh specimens. These may subsequently be frozen for rapid frozen section diagnosis.

Alternatively, 10% neutral buffered formalin may be used as a fixative for routine processing of larger tissue samples (i.e. post mortem specimens) into paraffin blocks. Subsequent processing protocols employ long processing times, to facilitate complete dehydration and infiltration of paraffin into the myelin.

It is important to note that brain, spinal and nerve tissue may contain transmissible spongiform encephalopathies (TSE) or prion diseases, which are neurodegenerative diseases that can affect humans and a variety of domestic and wild animal species. Prions are the causative agent of Creutzfeldt-Jakob disease in humans. The resulting holes in the brain tissue are remarkable (Fig 35). These infective prion agents are not inactivated by 10% formalin, so they remain potentially infectious, even after routine processing into paraffin. Formalin-fixed and paraffin-embedded tissues, especially of the brain, remain infectious. Treatment of formalin-fixed tissues from suspected cases for 30 min in 96% formic acid or phenol before histopathologic processing is considered to inactivate the prions, but such treatment may severely distort the microscopic neuropathology.

The safest method for ensuring that there is no risk of residual infectivity on contaminated instruments and other materials is to discard and destroy them by incineration.

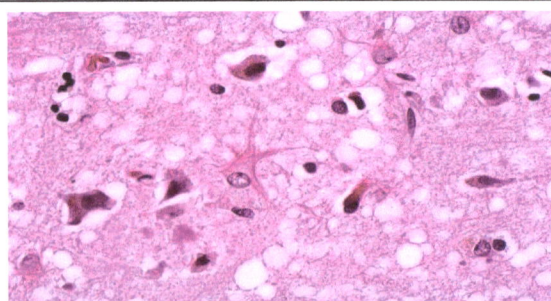

Fig 35. Crutzfeld-Jacob Disease showing spongiform change.

Bar Code Tracking in Histology

Specimen volumes continue to increase in both hospital and private pathology histology laboratories. Histology laboratories must adopt new procedures and strategies for managing this increasing volume of specimens to ensure the highest quality of patient care. Integration of new equipment and technologies for better management of all histology specimens is crucial.

Within the hospital pathology laboratory a standard protocol is to make certain to never assign consecutive accession numbers to the same tissue type. That is, the accessioning department would accession a skin specimen, then perhaps a liver specimen, before accessioning another skin specimen. This is the first in a long line of procedures developed to maintain specimen integrity from specimen receipt through final sign out of the report – a built in "double check" mechanism.

Private laboratories may not have this option. Usually, the majority, if not all, of the specimens are skin tissue in a dermatopathology laboratory. Therefore, it is the rule, rather than the exception, that there are many skin specimens accessioned consecutively. The integration and utilization of a bar code tracking system is one method of helping to ensure 100% accuracy in specimen identification.

The first opportunity for a unique specimen checkpoint is during the accessioning of the specimen. During accessioning, a unique two dimensional (2D) bar code label is affixed to (1) the specimen requisition, (2) the specimen bottles, and (3) each specimen cassette. When the surgical grossing process begins, the first step is to scan the 2D bar code on the requisition, the specimen bottle and the cassette. The information must match on all three items. If it does not, the laboratory information system (LIS) will not allow the grossing technician to continue. This procedure insures 100% accuracy with regard to the identity of the tissue within the cassette.

When used in conjunction with a bar coding identification / tracking system, the information from standardized surgical grossing techniques can be used to help maintain specimen integrity. During accessioning and grossing, patient and specimen information, in the form of a 2D bar code, are applied to the requisition and grossing cassette. Tissue processing cassettes are then placed into the tissue processor.

After processing, during the embedding phase, each cassette is removed one at a time from the holding well. The 2D bar code on the cassette is scanned, and the case information appears on the screen of the LIS. This information includes the gross description of the specimen type, along with the number of pieces of tissue in the cassette. Having access to this information is critically important to the embedding histologist. The information in the LIS can be double checked against exactly what is in the cassette, with regard to number of tissue pieces and specimen type. This step guarantees 100% accuracy of the specimen information at the embedding phase.

After the embedding is completed, the solidified blocks are taken out of the embedding molds, and any excess paraffin is removed from the block. This step is documented by scanning the 2D bar code on the block, and indicates that the blocks are now on a cold tray, in a refrigerator, waiting for microtomy.

The microtomy phase begins when a histologist removes a cold tray, containing blocks, from the refrigerator and takes it to their microtomy work station. The microtomy work station is standardized, and each histologist must follow the block cutting procedure exactly. Workflow is unidirectional; a block designated for cutting moves in only one direction, into and out of the microtome cutting area. In addition to the unidirectional workflow, the only labelled slides present in the work envelope are those for the block that is being cut.

Scanning the 2D bar code on the block time stamps the block as being "cut". It also provides the histologist with the case information in the LIS, which is used to generate a unique slide label, which also contains the 2D bar code. The scans in the microtomy phase provide two additional check points to ensure specimen integrity, and "one piece' work flow.

The block is cut into paraffin sections which are picked up on the corresponding microscope slide. Once a block is cut, it moves into the "block done" box – never back to the "block to be cut" area. The slides are placed into the "slides done" rack and moved into the oven for heating in order to remove water and melt the paraffin, thereby attaching the sections to the slides. When this microtomy procedure is followed, it ensures 100% accuracy with regard to the cut tissue matching the slide label information. Accidental "switching" of slides is not possible. The block is now logged as being "cut" in the LIS system.

Racks of mounted and baked slides for routine hematoxylin and eosin (H&E) staining are brought to the H&E slide staining area. After staining and coverslipping, each slide is visually inspected and checked against the corresponding block to provide a final check on specimen accuracy. The 2D bar code on the slide is scanned to indicate "slide checked". Additionally, slides are checked for H&E stain quality, and the results documented on a log sheet. Specifically, nuclei must appear blue with chromatin material visible, with eosin staining in the cytoplasm resulting in three shades of pink. The slides can now be brought to the office area for interpretation by the pathologist.

In summary, constant vigilance is required in the histology laboratory in order to guarantee specimen integrity. This vigilance can be enhanced to a greater degree by using a bar code tracking system. This Bar code tracking technology is recommended by the College of American Pathologists and the National Society for Histotechnology. In combination, bar code tracking and human diligence can result in an increase in patient care quality – a goal that all laboratorians should strive for.

Tissue Processing

Tissue processing begins with fixation. The fixative of choice in most histology laboratories is 10% neutral buffered formaldehyde (NBF). That is: this solution is made by diluting stock formaldehyde to a 10% concentration with phosphate buffer in the pH range of 7.0 to 7.4. Since stock formaldehyde is actually a 40% solution, the final chemical concentration of formaldehyde used in fixation is 4% formaldehyde.

Formaldehyde fixes tissue by crosslinking the proteins present. Fixation times will vary, depending upon tissue type and size. The general "rule of thumb" is to prepare tissue such that it is no thicker than 2 mm (i.e. the thickness of a nickel), and it should be in a specimen jar containing formaldehyde equaling 25 times the volume of the tissue. It should be noted that extended periods of fixation may alter antigenicity of proteins and inhibit enzymes. Conversely, if tissue is not fixed long enough, subsequent processing may cause artefacts such as "bubbling nuclei", which result when nuclei begin the fixation process in formaldehyde – but finish the process in alcohol, which "twists' the nuclear material within cells, causing the bubbling artefact.

Substitute fixatives for formaldehyde are available. Laboratories must be certain to validate any substitutes selected for fixation and processing, as the appearance and color balance in the final microscope slide may be affected. The subsequent standard tissue processing procedure dehydrates the tissue with alcohol, clears with xylene and infiltrates with molten paraffin wax. The tissues can then be embedded in paraffin to make blocks that can be cut on a microtome, generating sections to be affixed to microscope slides and stained. Substitutes can be made using different alcohols/ alcohol blends, xylene substitutes and varying blends of paraffin wax and polymers. The same validation rules apply as detailed above.

Standard tissue processing may be carried out on any number of open and closed tissue processors, although closed processors are preferred due to safety concerns, both for the tissues and laboratory personnel. Closed system processors are "smart' enough to prevent tissues from drying out in the event of a power failure, and the chemical fumes are kept inside the processor; released through filters and/or vented to the outside of the laboratory space.

Another tissue processing option is the use of microwave assisted processors that use conventional heat and microwaves to adjust and maintain temperature control during processing. Specimens are dehydrated through ethanol and isopropanol. Then, after vacuum vaporization, specimens are infiltrated with molten paraffin. The specimens are then ready for embedding. There are also ancillary units that will perform automated embedding of the tissues, if the proper cassettes are used.

A major advantage of microwave assisted tissue processors is the rapidity of processing of biopsy specimens. Small tissue biopsies of skin, prostate and gastrointestinal tissue can be processed into paraffin in approximately one hour. This is extremely valuable for cases requiring "rush" status. Another advantage is that, since no xylene is used, the tissues are generally much softer in the paraffin block, and therefore much easier to cut during microtomy, resulting in fewer cutting artefacts.

Processing procedures using microwave assisted tissue processors must be clearly and accurately defined, with much attention during the validation process. The fixation and dehydration steps must be complete to ensure proper infiltration with molten paraffin. Like routine tissue processors, the basic stages of tissue processing must accomplish:
   (a) Fixation of tissue to stabilize proteins and harden the tissue.
   (b) Dehydration of tissue to remove all unbound water.
   (c) Clearing of tissues to remove the dehydrant
   (d) Infiltration of tissue with molten paraffin, to ensure the embedding process is
       successful.

There are many factors involved in tissue processing, which provide many opportunities for things to go awry. Carry over of fixative into the processing alcohol can inhibit subsequent dehydration. If the absolute alcohol stations prior to the clearing stations contain water, this will result in incomplete dehydration as well. When water is left in the specimen, it cannot be removed by the clearant, and becomes trapped within the tissue during paraffin infiltration. The resulting paraffin blocks will be soft and difficult to cut during microtomy.

Conversely, tissue can become "over dehydrated" if the processing times in alcohol are too long. Tissues contain an amount of "bound water' within the nuclei and some other tissue elements. If this water is removed during extended dehydration, the resulting paraffin blocks may be dry / scratchy / hard to cut during microtomy. Soaking in cold ice water, once the block is faced off, may sometimes be used as a remedy. This is common in laboratories that use only one tissue processor to process all of their tissues, regardless of size and type. In this case, smaller tissues (i.e. biopsies) may become dry and brittle for cutting.

Processing Artefacts

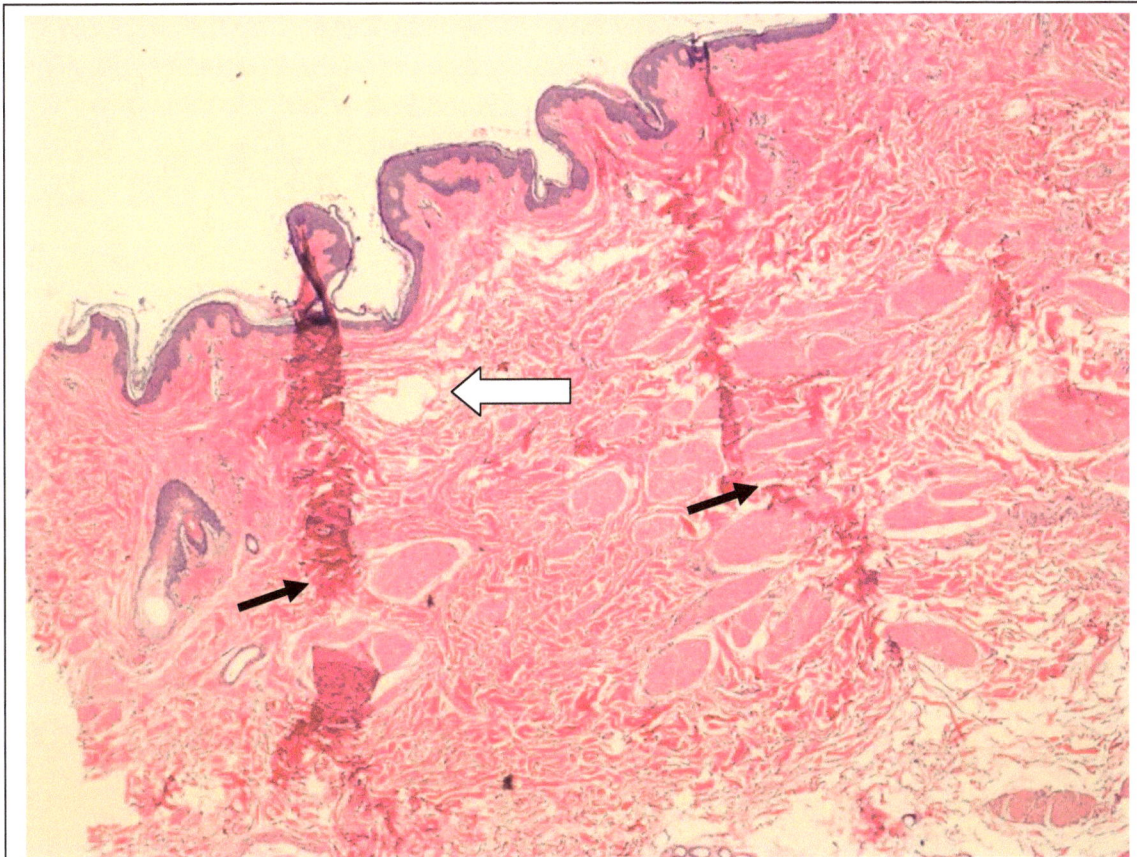

Figure 36. Skin specimen stained with H&E, original magnification x4
Hole/ tear: open arrow.   Folds/ wrinkles: closed arrows.

The most noticeable artefacts in Figure 36 are the wrinkles in the tissue sections (closed arrows). In addition, there are multiple holes and tears throughout the section (open arrow). Incomplete fixation would not cause such artefacts, as the cellular histology is acceptable (i.e. nuclear and cytoplasmic staining is with quality control limits). Improper embedding would also not be the cause of these artefacts. When skin specimens are mis-embedded, usually tearing and wrinkles would be localized within the epidermis, and within the dermal-epidermal junction.

The most likely cause of the artefacts seen in Figure 36 is a combination of incomplete dehydration, resulting in incomplete paraffin infiltration. When tissue is not completely dehydrated, excess water is left in the tissue. If xylene is used as the clearing agent, it can dissolve up to 2% water – but no more.   Also, if xylene substitutes are used, they are completely intolerant of any residual water. If water is present in the tissue after dehydration and clearing, paraffin cannot infiltrate the tissue completely. Without complete paraffin infiltration, the tissue can tear and fold during microtomy. If this affects all tissues in the run, the tissues may have to be reprocessed by melting down the blocks and placing the tissues back into the cassettes, with new cassette tops. The cassettes can now be run back through changes of xylene and 100% alcohol. After rinsing in 95% alcohol, the tissues can be put back onto the tissue processor to begin processing at the formalin step. Finally, they can be run back through xylene and into paraffin. This procedure should remedy the problem.

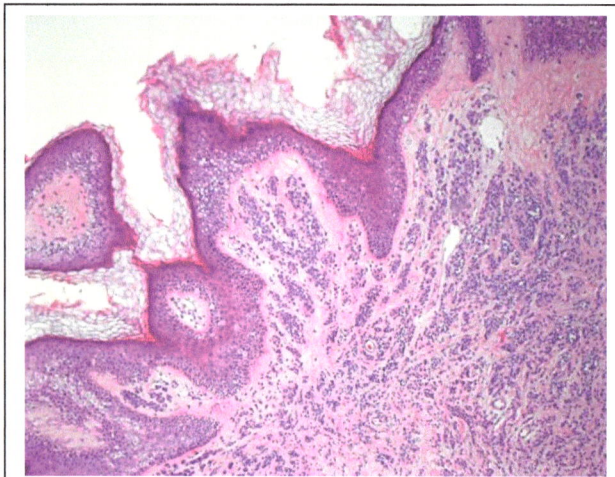

Figure 37. Skin specimen, H&E, original magnification x10

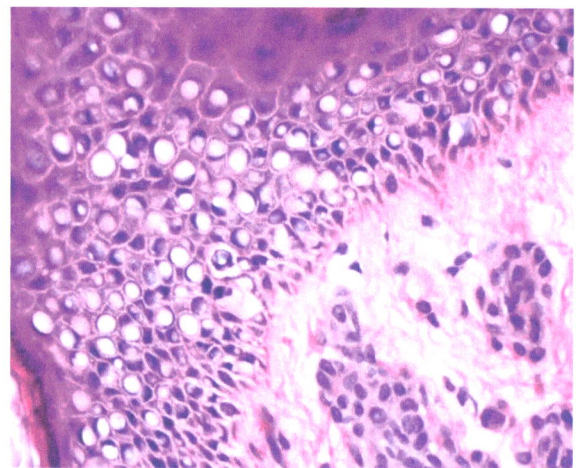

Figure 38. Skin specimen, H&E, original magnification x40

Can you spot the artefact shown in Figures 37 and 38?
Under both low and high power magnification, one can observe vacuolization of many cells, sometimes referred to as the "swiss cheese effect". These large, empty circular spaces are located within cells, and show some nuclei to be pushed to one side of the cell. This is an artefact sometimes seen in northern latitudes, as it is caused by slow freezing of the tissue specimen. During this slow freezing process, ice crystals can form within the cell. As we all know, when water changes to ice, it expands and takes up more space. These ice crystals are the cause of the resulting empty spaces within the cell.

This artefact is not observed in the "rapid freezing" of fresh tissue in a cryostat. The tissue should be frozen so quickly, that ice crystals do not have an opportunity to form. If you are observing this artefact in your cryostat sections, the tissue is not being frozen rapidly enough.

Reference laboratories operating in northern climates can help to prevent this artefact by providing formalin fixative that contains up to 10% ethanol. Addition of the ethanol helps to decrease the freezing point of the fixative/ tissue. It is not recommended to add ethanol in a percentage greater than 10%, as it may cause the tissue to exhibit "foamy nuclei" – bubbles within the nuclear material. This artefact results from the tissue undergoing fixation from both formaldehyde and ethanol at the same time. These chemicals have different fixation chemistry, which occur at different times, and can result in the "foamy nuclei" artefact.

Hematoxylin and Eosin Staining

The hematoxylin and eosin (H&E) stain is the standard procedure in any histology laboratory. The pathologist relies on formalin fixed, paraffin embedded H&E stained slides to determine diagnoses. While the H&E employs a standard protocol, individual laboratories produce slides of varying tinctorial color. Some factors that affect this stain are listed below.

- Hematoxylin. There are two major types of hematoxylin staining. A Harris' hematoxylin is used in "regressive" staining in which the sections are over-stained in hematoxylin and then differentiated in acid alcohol to selectively stain nuclei. Gill type hematoxylins are used in a "progressive" stain whereby the longer the sections are left in the hematoxylin, the darker the nuclei stain. Harris' hematoxylin will stain nuclei dark blue, while Gill hematoxylin results in a more purple hue. Hematoxylin is a natural dye obtained from the logwood tree *Haematoxylon campechianum* that will stain the nuclei of cells blue/black. The staining is enhanced by the addition of an aluminum, iron or lead salt, which acts as a mordant for the hematoxylin to bind to the tissue sites.

- Eosin. Use of alcoholic eosin solutions should result in three distinct shades of pink in the tissue section cytoplasm with red blood cells, loose connective tissue and compact connective tissue displaying the three colors. Phloxine may be added to the eosin solution to "brighten" the color rendition. Eosin staining may be followed by 95% alcohol, as this helps to differentiate the stain.

- Clarifier. The composition of this solution varies. The original procedure written by Lee Luna in the Armed Forces Institute of Pathology (AFIP) Manual specifies differentiation of the Harris hematoxylin solution with a "1% acid alcohol" solution for a time duration of "a few quick dips". This solution is 1% hydrochloric acid in 70% ethanol. However, with the current use of automated stainers, "a few quick dips" needs to be quantified into seconds or minutes. This usually requires a dilution of the original clarifier solution, with some experiments to determine the exact time. The recommended starting point for clarifier on an automated stainer is to use the following for 30 seconds:

100% ethanol	700 ml
tap water	2600 ml
hydrochloric acid (concentrated)	2.0 ml

Once made, the resulting intensity of the nuclear stain can be adjusted by changing the time of the clarifier incubation. Alternatively, one may adjust the amount of acid added to the alcohol (i.e. decrease from 2.0 ml to 1.5 ml). These adjustments will allow you to obtain a final stain with the required nuclear staining intensity.

- Bluing reagent. Several different solutions can be used as a "bluing" reagent. After staining with hematoxylin, and differentiation with clarifier, the nuclei in tissue sections is still reddish. The bluing reagent transforms this red color to a deep blue. The composition of these bluing reagent solutions varies. However, they all function in providing positive ions that bind to the hematoxylin to effect a color change from reddish to the final blue seen in the nuclei. Lithium carbonate and dilute ammonium hydroxide are specified as bluing reagents. In fact, warm tap water may also be used to "blue" sections as well. It is important that the pH of the bluing reagent is not too high, as section loss may occur during staining. The recommended starting point for bluing reagent is:

Bluing reagent:	
Tap water	3500 ml
Ammonium hydroxide (concentrated)	1.5 ml

As with the clarifier solution, results can be obtained by adjusting the time of incubation and/or concentration of the solution. Alternatively, one can use lithium carbonate as a bluing reagent, or simply use a running water step to "blue" the nuclei.

- Eosin. Working eosin solution is the most stable reagent of the H&E stain. Hundreds of slides can be stained with the same batch of eosin on board an automated stainer. The incubation time is usually kept short, as eosin penetrates and stains rapidly and reproducibly (i.e. 1-2 minutes). The variable step in eosin staining is the subsequent 95% alcohol incubation, which produces the final "three shades of pink" within the tissue sections. The number of 95% stations (i.e. one or two), and the incubation times (i.e. 30 seconds to 2 minutes) will determine the final quality of eosin staining. Finally, it is important that the final 100% alcohol stations after the eosin staining remain uncontaminated with water. Any water left in the sections after the coverslip is applied may cause the eosin to "bleed out" of the section.

Complete removal of paraffin is an essential first step in any H&E staining procedure. If xylene substitutes are being used, it may be necessary to adjust and lengthen times to guarantee paraffin removal. In addition, xylene substitutes do not tolerate traces of water, as xylene does. Thus, it is important also in the dehydration steps prior to coverslipping that the slides move through fresh changes of alcohol and xylene substitute. If any water remains in the sections during coverslipping, the final slides will appear cloudy. Additionally, the eosin stain may bleed out of the sections.

A standard H&E staining protocol is provided in the Procedures section. While it may not be ideal for your laboratory, it can be used as a starting point. The final color rendition of your H&E stain should be determined by working with your pathologists. This will consequently make their job easier. Each day, once the H&E stain set up is completed, you should run down one test slide to confirm that the staining is optimal. This also will help you to document quality control procedures.

Mucin Stains

Introduction

When staining sections for the presence of carbohydrates, the two main classes under investigation are glycogen and mucins. Mucins include substances referred to as mucopolysaccharides, mucosubstances, glycoproteins and glycoconjugates.

Mucins provide an environment that is conducive to molecular diffusion of chemicals, especially those in ionic form. Mucin also increases the binding between cells, and may help to "shed' bacteria and viruses. The demonstration of the presence and absence of mucins within tissue sections is an important tool to assist pathologists in rendering a diagnosis. The following types of mucins can be distinguished by certain special stains.

Acidic mucins contain sulphur in varying amounts. Other acidic mucins can have carboxyl groups attached to them, which make them acidic.

Neutral mucins, as the name implies, contain no acidic reactive groups within. These mucins are epithelial in origin and are commonly found in gastric lining cells.

 Alcian blue is the most common stain used for demonstrating the presence of acidic mucins, since the blue dye molecules are cationic (positively charged) and bind to the anionic sulphur and carboxyl groups within the mucin. Neutral mucins are not usually stained by alcian blue. The pH of the alcian blue solution can be adjusted to stain different classes of acidic mucins (Figure 39A and 39B). Alcian blue can also be combined with a PAS stain to show both acidic and neutral mucins (Figure 40). Mucicarmine is sometimes used to demonstrate acidic mucins (Figure 41). Mucicarmine also will stain encapsulated fungi such as *Cyrptococcus neoformans.*

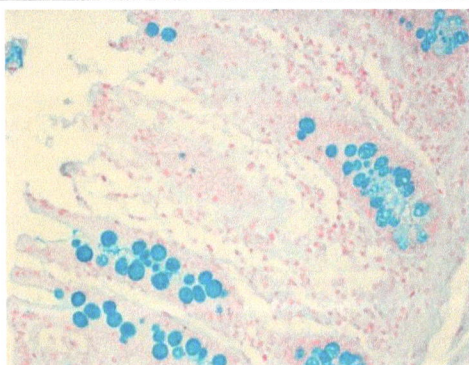

Figure 39A. Alcian Blue pH 1.0
Original magnification x400

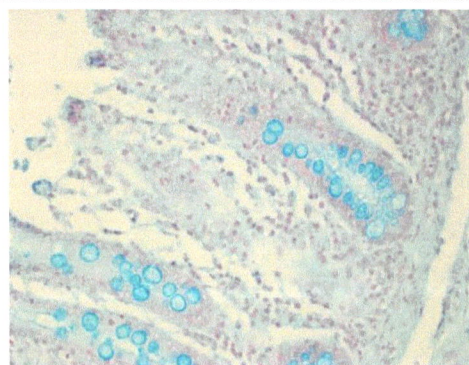

Figure 39B. Alcian Blue pH 2.5
Original magnification x400

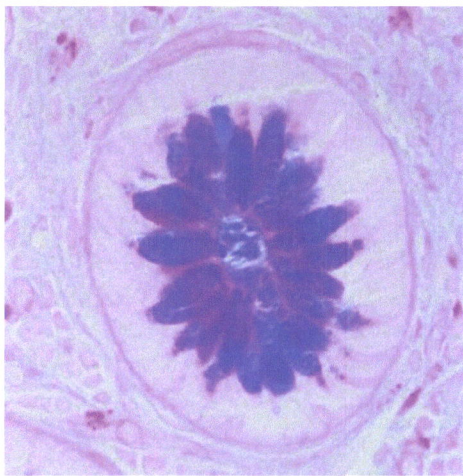

Figure 40. Alcian Blue / PAS
Original magnification x600

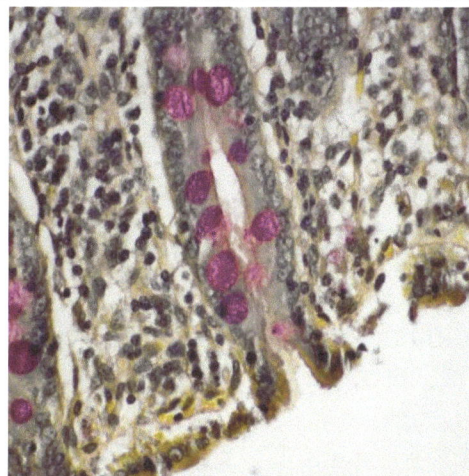

Figure 41. Mucicarmine
Original magnification x600

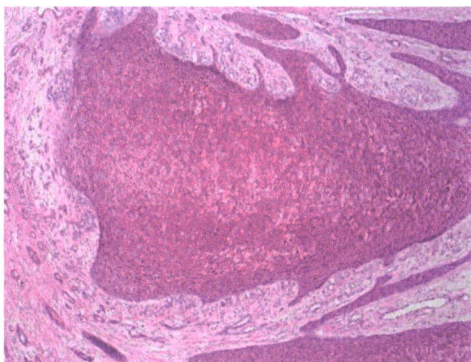

Figure 42A. PAS
For glycogen
Original magnification x100

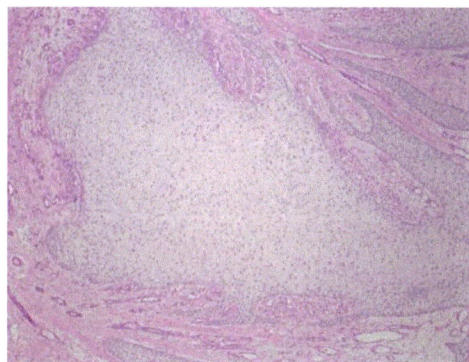

Figure 42B. PAS + D
For glycogen
Original magnification x100

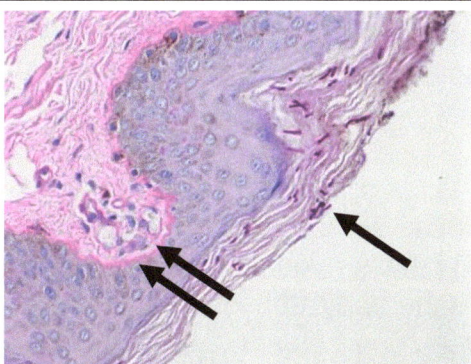

Figure 43A. PAS for fungi in skin
(single arrow) and basement
membrane (double arrow)
Original magnification x400

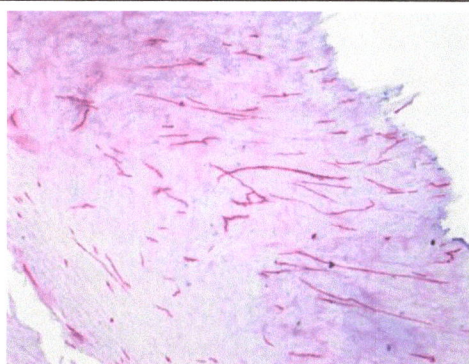

Figure 43B. PAS
For fungi in nail specimen
Original magnification x600

Glycogen is the cellular mode of storing sugar, which is in the form of a six-sided molecule. Glycogen can be demonstrated histologically using the periodic acid – Schiff's stain (PAS). The glycogen molecules are oxidized by the periodic acid, which breaks the ring and exposes aldehyde groups. Subsequent exposure to Schiff's reagent causes the aldehyde groups to react with it and form a pink reaction product (Figure 42A).

Presence of glycogen is confirmed by staining a serial section of the tissue with periodic acid – Schiff's plus diastase (PAS+D). The section is incubated with diastase solution prior to performing the PAS stain – in order to digest all of the glycogen. The end result is the absence of pink stain (Figure 42B).

It is important to remember that the Schiff's stain is not specific for glycogen. Schiff's reagent will combine with any aldehyde groups to form pink reaction product. This is evident in using the PAS stain to identify the basement membrane in skin specimens (Figure 43A). Additionally, the PAS stain can be used to stain fungi (Figure 43A, 43B). The sugars present in the basement membrane and the fungal cell wall are oxidized and react with the Schiff's reagent to form the pink reaction product. Digestion with diastase does not remove the staining.

Fungi include molds, yeasts and higher fungi. All fungi are eukaryotic and have sterols but not peptidoglycan in their cell membrane. Their cell walls are composed of cellulose; the same building blocks that plants use. Fungi may produce large, reproductive mycelium, called mushrooms, which may be edible, or poisonous. Other naturally occurring fungi may infect humans and cause skin infections, sometimes known as "athlete's foot".

Fungi are chemoheterotrophs which require organic nutrition and most are aerobic. Many fungi are also saprophytes which live off of dead organic matter, in soil and water and acquire their food by absorption. Fungi may produce sexual and asexual spores. There are over 100,000 species recognized, with over 100 of them known to be infectious agents in humans. Molds are composed of numerous, microscopic, branching hyphae known collectively as a mycelium.

Hyphae growth occurs from the apical tip, and apical vesicles contain materials and enzymes for the formation of new hyphal wall. Older hyphae are less biochemically active and contain many storage vacuoles. In most molds these hyphae have septa, which are cross-walled divisions, but in some there are none and the hyphae are aseptate. A septum is a cross-wall formation which divides one fungal hypha into two cells. These septa may add strength to the hyphae or serve to isolate adjacent parts to allow differentiation, such as during production of the reproductive structures.

Spores are formed from the reproductive mycelium. Asexual spores are produced by the aerial mycelium of a single organism, whereas sexual spores are formed by the fusion of cells and nuclei from opposite mating strains (Figures 44 and 45).

Fungal nail infections are common infections of the fingernails or toenails that can cause the nail to become discolored, thick, and more likely to crack and break. [1]The technical name for a fungal nail infection is "onychomycosis."

Fungal nail infections can be caused by many different types of fungi (yeasts or molds) that live in the environment. Small cracks in your nail or the surrounding skin can allow these germs to enter your nail and cause an infection. A diagnosis of onychomycosis can be made by taking a nail clipping to look at under a microscope or send to a laboratory for a fungal culture.

Your histology laboratory may receive skin and nail specimens to be evaluated for presence of fungi. The most common special stains used to visualize fungi are the periodic acid Schiff's stain (PAS) and the Grocott's methenamine silver stain for fungi (GMS).

Both stains are based on the chemistry of the fungal cell wall, which is made of cellulose. Cellulose is composed of glucose molecules, attached together very tightly. The PAS stain uses a primary step of oxidation of the glucose with periodic acid to form aldehyde groups. Once formed, the aldehydes are available to subsequently bind with the Schiff's reagent, which results in the fungal cell walls being stained pink (Figure 46). Diastase digestion may, or may not be used, as it does not affect the fungal staining; it simply removes any glycogen which may be present.

Some dermatopathologists feel that the GMS stain is a more sensitive stain for detection of fungi in tissue sections. In this stain, chromic acid is used to oxidize the glucose molecules, leaving the aldehyde groups open to bind silver molecules, present in the methenamine silver solution. Subsequent development and toning of the sections renders the fungal cell walls black (Figure 47).

Either the PAS or the GMS method may be utilized to stain fungi in tissue sections. The previous section on Hair Histology describes how to stain fungi that are present on hair shafts.

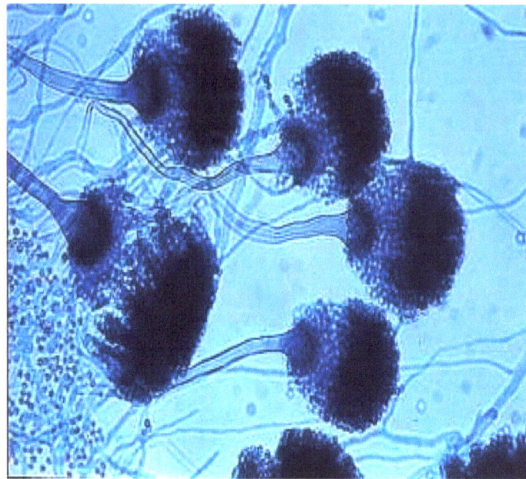

Figure 44. Aspergillus conidia.
Macroscopic view.

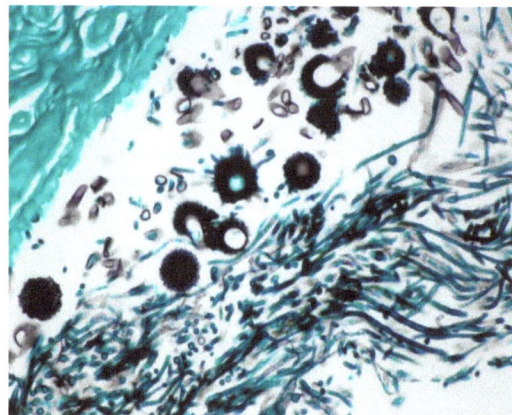

Figure 45. GMS stain showing fungal
hyphae and conidia stained black.
Original magnification x200.

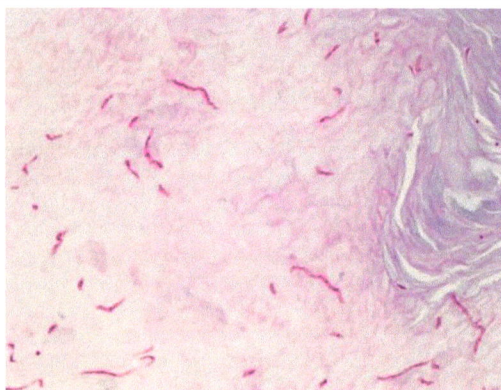

Figure 46. Fungal hyphae stained
pink with the PAS stain.
Original magnification x200.

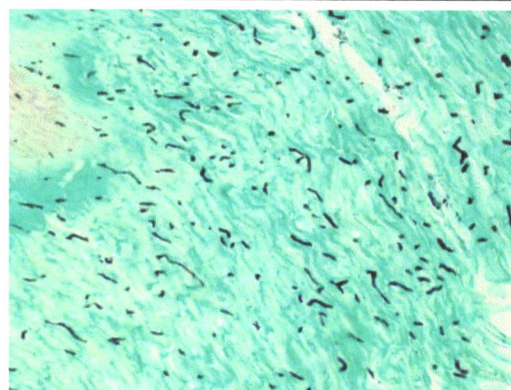

Figure 47. Fungal hyphae stained
black with the GMS stain.
Original magnification x200.

Microorganism Stains

The staining of microorganisms in histology can be challenging. Filamentous fungi and associated conidia are more easily demonstrated as they are visible under light microscopy when stained with periodic acid Schiff's (PAS) as in Figure 48. The diameter of fungi filaments is 5-10 microns, which is approximately the same as the diameter of a red blood cell, while their length may be hundreds of microns (Figure 49). Microorganisms are extremely small and are at the limit of resolution of the light microscope. Viruses are even smaller (Figure 50).

Bacteria exist in three different shapes. Cocci are round, bacilli appear as rods and spirochetes are corkscrew shaped. The first level of determination for bacteria is whether they are Gram positive or Gram negative. The original method of Gram's technique published in 1884 is still used today. Tissue sections are first stained with a crystal violet solution, which stains all of the tissue section. This is followed by Gram's iodine which locks the crystal violet stain into the cell wall of the bacteria. Subsequent decolorization with acetone removes the stain from everything – except the Gram "positive" bacteria, which remain a dark blue/purple color (Figure 51).

The second phase of the stain involves the application of fuchsin / neutral red solution which stains Gram "negative" bacteria pink/red (Figure 52). This can be the most variable step in the procedure and relies on the correct application and retention of the basic fuchsin within Gram negative bacteria.

There are two additional steps which may result in variable staining as well. The first is an over-decolorization with acetone, which may result in faint staining of Gram positive bacteria. The second is the use and timing of the final counterstain, which may be either picric acid/acetone or tartrazine. While picric acid/acetone results in a more reliable result, the picric acid is a dangerous chemical and requires specific disposal procedures. Tartrazine is safer, but can easily be leached out during the dehydration process prior to coverslipping. The histotechnician performing this stain must rely on experience and precise timing to produce consistent results for this stain.

Actinomycetes are a Gram positive, non-acid fast, branching filamentous organism. However, care must be taken when performing the Gram positive stain sequence. It may be necessary to (a) increase the time in crystal violet solution and (b) decrease the time in the acetone decolorization step in order to demonstrate the organism.

A second determination of bacteria is based on an organisms "acid fastness". The Kinyoun method for acid fast bacteria, the Fite method for leprosy bacilli and the Ziehl-Neelsen stain for tubercule bacilli are all based on the same stain theory. Tissue sections are first stained with a carbol fuchsin solution, which stains all tissue elements pink/red. Subsequent decolorization in an acid-alcohol solution removes stain from all the tissue elements, except acid fast bacteria. Methylene blue is usually used as a counterstain (Figure 53).

Spirochete bacteria are ubiquitous in nature. They are found everywhere in soil and water. The issue is that some are pathogenic to humans. The *Treponema pallidum* spirochete is sexually transmitted and causes syphilis. The *Borrelia burgdorferi* spirochete is present in certain tick species, and may be transmitted to humans when the tick attaches to the skin to feed. The result is Lyme disease, which if left untreated, can be debilitating to the patient.

Silver stains were developed in the early 1900's to stain spirochetes. The Dieterle (1927), Warthin-Starry (1920) and Steiner (1944) are still used in histology today to demonstrate spirochetes. Some of the methods have been modified to make them safer to use (Margeson and Chapman, 1996). The stain theory is the same in all methods: pre-treat the sections to make the spirochetes more readily able to pick up and bind the silver solution. The final result is to stain the spirochetes black, against a gray/ brown background (Figure 54). Those who have performed any of these stains are aware of the many staining procedure pitfalls, which can render the spirochetes either over or under stained.   As a result, many laboratories currently use immunohistochemistry to stain spirochetes. While both methods can stain spirochetes, neither is able to demonstrate the exact species to which the stained organism belongs.

Both positive and negative control slides should be used when performing stains for microorganisms. The negative control slide ensures that there is no bacterial contamination present in source water or stain solutions.

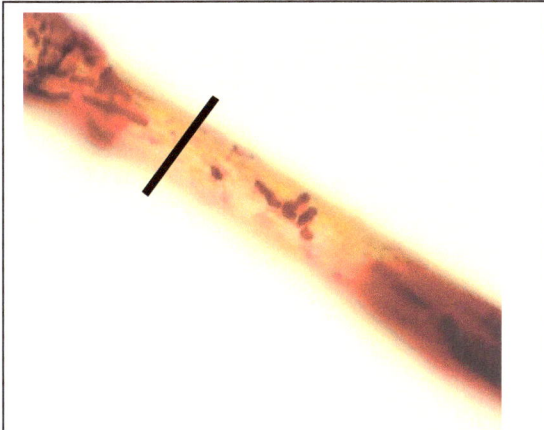

Figure 48. PAS stain on human hair showing red fungi (10 micron diameter). Bar shows 100 microns.

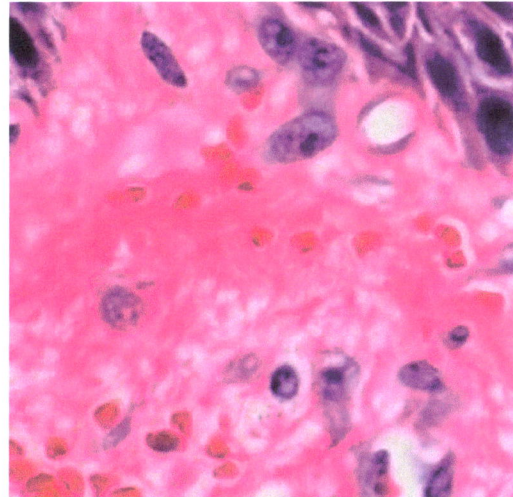

Figure 49. Red blood cells (pink, 8 microns) and cell nuclei (blue, 20 microns).

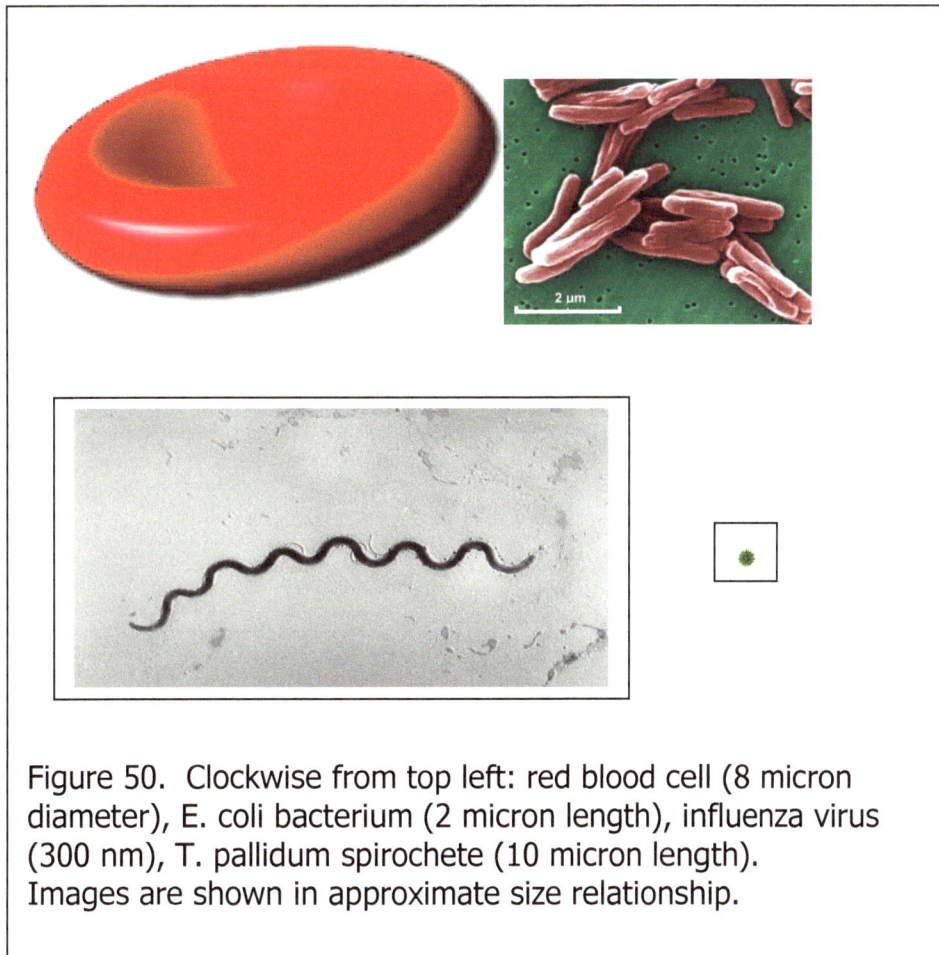

Figure 50. Clockwise from top left: red blood cell (8 micron diameter), E. coli bacterium (2 micron length), influenza virus (300 nm), T. pallidum spirochete (10 micron length).
Images are shown in approximate size relationship.

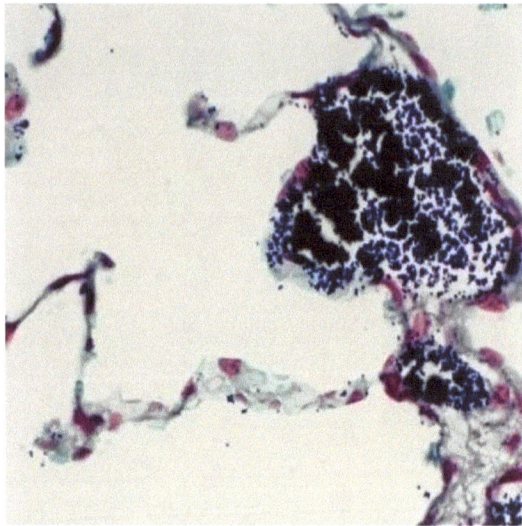

Figure 51. Gram positive bacteria, dark blue.
Original magnification x 600

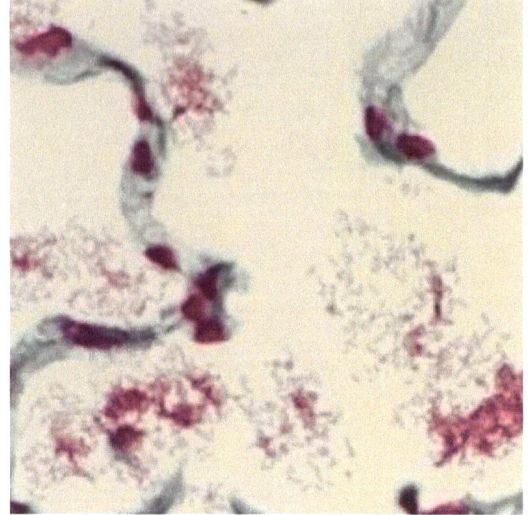

Figure 52. Gram negative bacteria, small red clumps.
Original magnification x 600

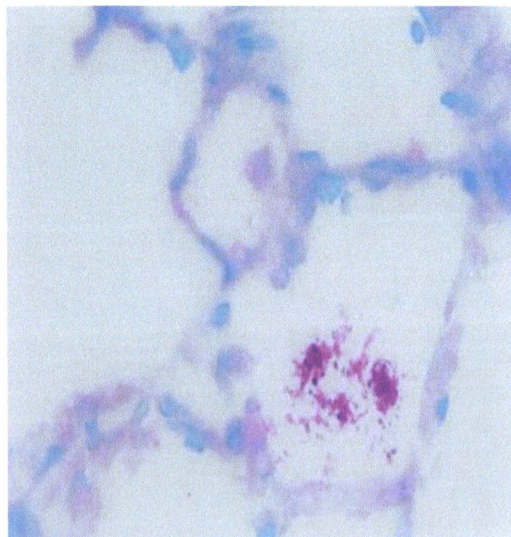

Figure 53. Leprosy bacilli, dark red clump.
Original magnification x 600

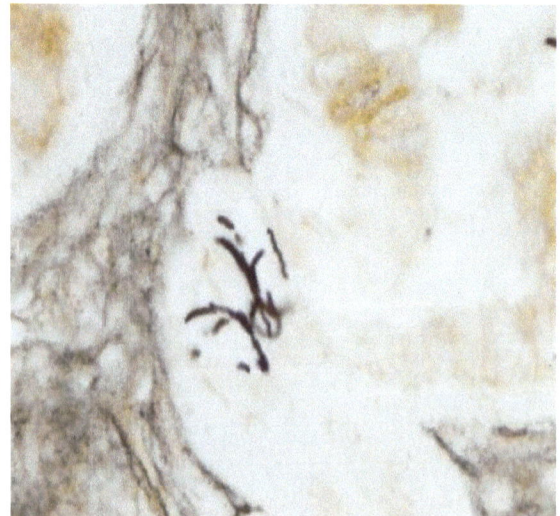

Figure 54. Spirochetes, dark black, corkscrew shaped.
Original magnification x 600

Silver Stains

In the histology world, the mere mention of a "silver stain" may be the cause of panic and uncertainty with regard to the performance of the stain, and the quality of the final resulting microscope slide. All other special stains, with few exceptions, are relatively easy and straightforward to perform; not so with silver stains.

Silver stains can be categorized into (a) stains to visualize substances, such as calcium, melanin and reticulin and (b) stains for microorganisms, such as fungi and spirochetes. The goal of all silver stains is the same: to get metallic silver to precipitate out at the staining site, and then replace it with gold to provide the final, stabilized, black reaction product.

Silver stains were developed in the early 1900's to stain spirochetes. The Dieterle (1927), Warthin-Starry (1920) and Steiner (1944) are still used in histology today to demonstrate spirochetes. Some of the methods have been modified to make them safer to use (Margeson and Chapman, 1996).

The specific procedures for these stains are outside of the scope of this discussion. However, the following stain procedure outline explains the steps used.

<u>Oxidation</u> enhances subsequent staining by the silver solution. Oxidizers include phosphomolybdic acid, potassium permanganate and periodic acid.

<u>Sensitization</u> usually employs a metal salt to help bind silver from the silver solution. The original sensitizer for Wilder's silver technique and the Steiner and Steiner stain is 1% uranyl nitrate. However, Margeson and Chapman (1996) pioneered the substitution of zinc formalin for the original radioactive uranyl nitrate solution, which is also a strong oxidizer, and considered hazardous.

<u>Silver impregnation solution</u> contains metallic silver in a solution. The idea is to have the silver carrying solution composed such that the silver ions will move from the solution, bind to the tissue section and then precipitate out in metallic form.

The <u>reduction</u> step in the reaction involves providing electrons, in the form of substances such as hydroquinone and formaldehyde, to chemically make the silver ions precipitate out into visible metallic silver. This allows the structures in question to be visualized in dark black staining.

<u>Toning</u> of the sections in gold chloride is a chemical reaction whereby the metallic silver is replaced by metallic gold, which is very stable and maintains the black color product.

The use of sodium thiosulfate, or "hypo", helps to remove any unbound silver remaining from the toning reaction. This is followed by counterstaining, usually either with nuclear fast red or fast green, for a proper final color rendition.

Thus, with all of these simple, straight forward steps, what could possibly go wrong? Let's begin at the beginning and work it through.

<u>Use acid clean glassware</u> for all containers and Coplin jars. Why? This will prevent the presence of any unwanted ions on the glass surfaces (including the slides themselves) causing non- specific precipitation of the silver. You will see this as a black/ or mirror precipitate on the inside of the Coplin jar, or on the surface of the microscope slide. If this does happen, the unwanted silver can be removed (see Procedure section).

<u>Use plastic forceps</u> to handle all slides --- not metal. Metal present in metal forceps may cause the silver to precipitate out. Back in the old days, before plastic forceps, we simply dipped the tines of metal forceps into paraffin, allowed it to cool, thereby preventing the metal from contacting any of the solutions.

<u>Pay attention</u> to the slides when they are in the silver solution – especially if the solution is a hot, heated solution. The point at which the silver solution itself may precipitate out is a fine one. The slides and staining solution should be monitored closely during these incubations. Also, if you are monitoring the slide under a microscope, make sure to rinse the slide in distilled water before viewing, thereby preventing black silver precipitate forming on the microscope stage. Your coworkers especially will appreciate this.

Microscope Use

As a histologist, you should be well versed in the proper installation, alignment and use of a compound light microscope (shown below).

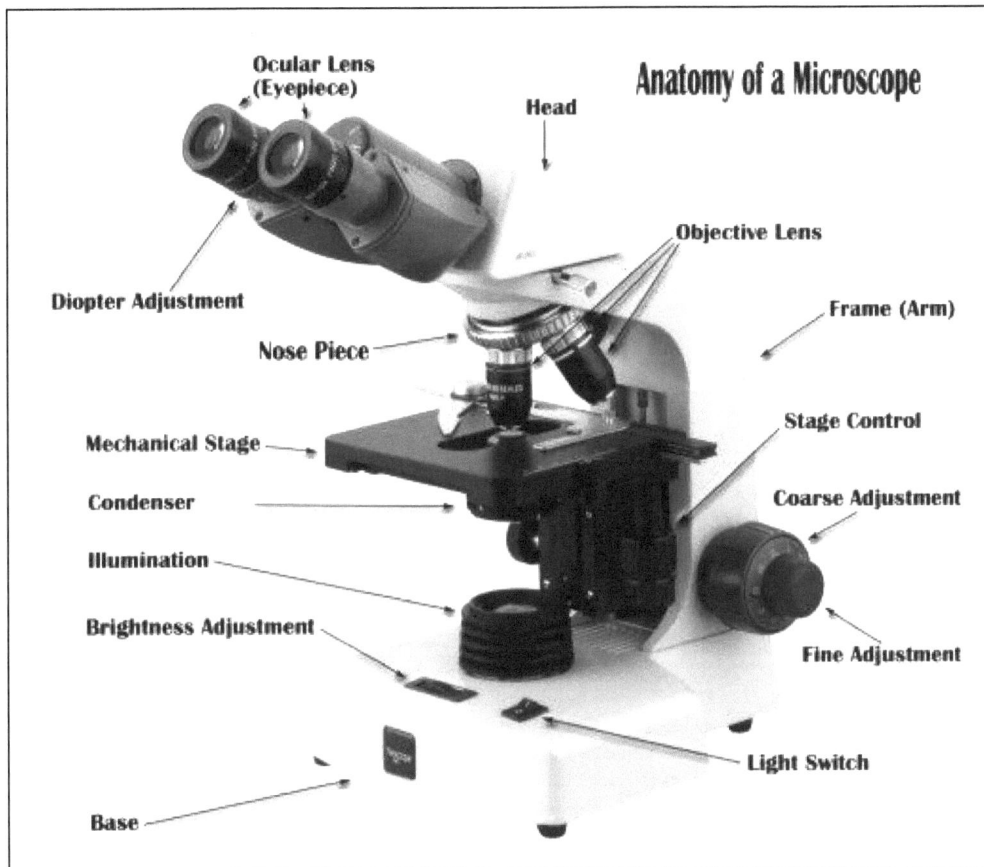

Anatomy of a Microscope

However, most histologists have not received proper instruction in this regard. It is very important that you know the proper "care and feeding" rules for your microscope. Only in this way will you be able to view optimal microscope images consistently. This is especially important for assessing routine hematoxylin and eosin (H&E), special and immunohistochemical stain quality.

Safety First

Anytime you have to move a microscope, you should have one hand under the base, and the other hand grasping the "arm" that holds the head. Make certain you have unplugged the microscope, and that the electrical cord is secured to the top of the microscope; not dragging on the floor where it can trip you. Once the microscope is set up, make certain the light intensity is on "low" each time you look into the oculars for the first time. High light intensity focused on your retina could cause damage. The microscope should be cleaned and maintained by a professional at least every six months to ensure proper operation (this is also a CLIA regulation). Finally, the microscope should undergo an annual 'electrical check" to ensure safety from electrical shock (this is also CAP checklist item).

<u>Microscope Alignment</u>
Every time that you sit down at a microscope, you should follow the alignment procedure outlined below.

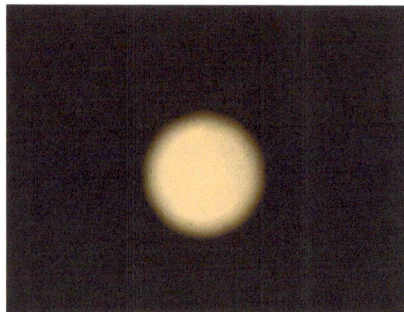

Figure 55. Close down illumination ring.

Figure 56. Move condenser up/down to obtain sharp image.

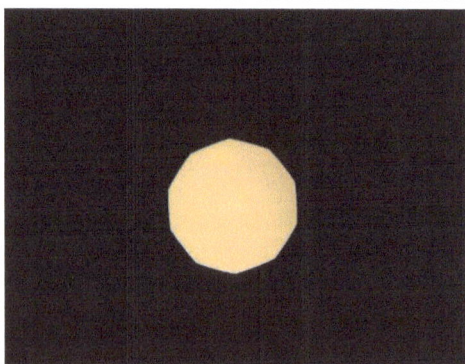

Figure 57. Center the condenser.

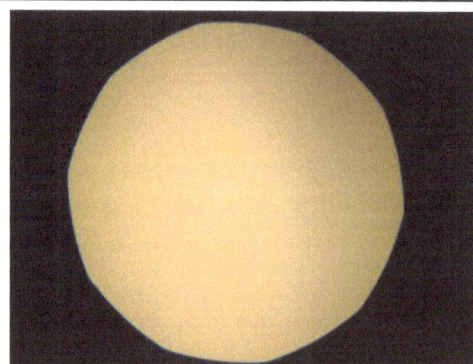

Figure 58. Open condenser.

Alignment Procedure

1. Make sure the power cord is plugged in. Turn on the light switch. Adjust brightness to half way.
2. Look through the eyepiece (i.e. the oculars). Pull/push them until you see one light field with both your eyes.
3. Close down the illumination ring (Figure 55).
4. Move the condenser up/down until you get a sharp image (Figure 56).
5. Use the condenser X-Y adjustments to move the light field to the center (Figure 57).
6. Open up the illumination ring all the way. The light source is now centered (Figure 58).
7. Place a stained slide on the stage.
8. Move the 10x objective lens into position.
9. Look through the eye piece. Close/cover your left eye. Use the Coarse/Fine adjustment to obtain a sharp image of the slide.
10. Continue to look through the eyepiece. Close/cover your right eye. Use the Diopter Adjustment to focus the slide image.
11. You are now ready to look at slides.

Tips for Success

If you do not use a microscope frequently, or you have trouble looking with both eyes, simply cover one of your eyes with your hand (or close the eye) and view through one ocular. You may elect to use the mechanical stage, with controls – or simply move the slide with one hand, while using the other hand on the coarse and fine focus adjustment.

If you are using a multiple viewing microscope, with more than one eyepiece, the person "driving" should focus first. Then, additional personnel should bring the image into focus. Only in that way will everyone be in the same plane of focus. Usually, these microscopes are outfitted with an "arrow" as well, in order for the "driver" to point out areas of interest.

If you have a microscope designated for use in Special Stains, please make certain to clean off the stage after every viewing. Water, coverslipping mountant, etc. may spill onto the stage area while viewing.

Use the coarse adjustment only when the low power objective is in place. ***Never*** use the coarse adjustment at higher powers. Doing this may drive the condenser into the slide and break it, and/or damage the objective. Objective lenses are usually provided at 10x, 20X and 40X. Some microscopes may have a 4X and 100X high power objective as well. The high power objective should be designated as either "oil immersion" or "high dry".   The eyepiece usually contains oculars at 10X. To obtain the final magnification of the image you are viewing, simply multiply the ocular lens power by the objective lens power. For example, if you are viewing a slide through a 10X power ocular, using the 10X objective, the final magnification is 10 times 10 = 100X.

Do's and Don'ts for a light microscope:
DO carry a microscope with two hands: one hand gripping the Frame/Arm, the other under the base.
DO leave the lowest power objective in place when the microscope is not in use.
DON'T leave the light source on when you are done – turn off the light switch.

If you follow the above alignment procedure and tips for success, you will always have a safe, pleasant microscope viewing experience.

Immunohistochemistry Summary

There are some pathological conditions that exist that cannot be accurately diagnosed by examining hematoxylin and eosin (H&E) stained slides alone. In such cases, the pathologist may order immunohistochemical (IHC) stains to help render a diagnosis. Immunohistochemical stains are classified as either immunofluorescence (IF) or immunochromogen; however both make use of highly specific antibody preparations to detect their specific antigens in tissue sections. Direct immunofluorescence (DIF) utilizes a fluorescent label attached directly to the antibody. Upon viewing under ultraviolet (UV) light in a dark field microscope, the label fluoresces an apple green color (Figure 59, 60).

Immunofluorescence is further classified into direct immunofluorescence (DIF) or indirect immunofluorescence (IIF). This procedure is done for patients who present with bullous (i.e. blistering) disease, which may have an autoimmune cause. DIF is done by cutting frozen sections of the patient's skin specimen, and then incubating these slides with specific fluorescein labeled antibodies. IIF makes use of the patient's serum, serially diluted and incubated on substrate slides (i.e. frozen sections of monkey esophagus). A second fluorescein labeled antibody is then applied. The resulting slides of both DIF and IIF procedures are then viewed in a dark field fluorescence microscope and the pathologist records the resulting staining patterns to make an accurate diagnosis (Figure 61).

Immunochromogen stains are performed on sections of formalin fixed paraffin embedded tissue (i.e. the identical material from which the H&E slide is made from). Sections are cut, baked and then hydrated to stain either manually or with automated technology. The resulting specific chromogen stain can be viewed under regular light microscopy. Whether or not a particular antigen is present helps the pathologist to make an accurate diagnosis.

Immunochromogen (IC) methods are based on the same mechanism as immunofluorescence methods. Specific antibodies are used to detect and bind to specific antigens located within the tissue section. These antigens may be proteins located on the exterior of the cell, within the interior of the cell, on the cell membrane, on the nuclear membrane, or within the nucleus. There are even other, in situ methods, that can detect gene aberrations within the nucleus.

Antibodies themselves are too small to be seen under a microscope. So, like the IF procedures, the IC procedures employ methods to "label" the site of antibody: antigen binding. Figure 62 is a schematic representation of the IC method. The primary antibody binds to the antigen present in the tissue section. A secondary antibody, labeled with a link (either a biotin or polymer link) is applied, and binds to the primary antibody. The final detection molecules are added, and bind to the link reagents. These detection molecules form colored precipitates at the site of antibody binding when they are developed. Final reaction products can be brown, red or blue, depending upon the chromogen used (Figure 63).

An important detail is that specimens for DIF must be collected into a specific immunofluorescence transport medium, such as Michel's medium, in the clinicians' office. The specimens must then be recognized when they arrive in the histology laboratory and routed to the immunohistochemistry laboratory. ***At no time can these specimens be exposed to formaldehyde.*** Formaldehyde exposure renders these specimens unsuitable for immunofluorescence.

Detection of protein antigens within tissues and cells assists the pathologist in making accurate diagnoses. This is especially important when the diagnosis cannot be made entirely with the H&E slide. The results may also be used in determining how to treat the patient.

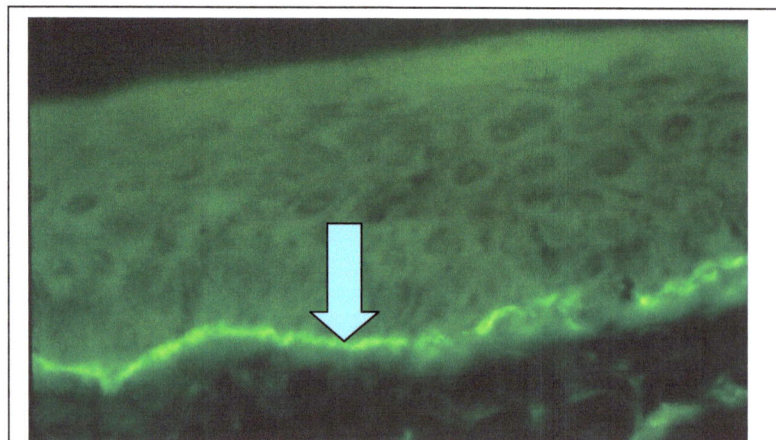

Figure 59. Postivie immunoflourescence is demonstrated at the dermal-epidermal junction (arrow). Original magnification x 600

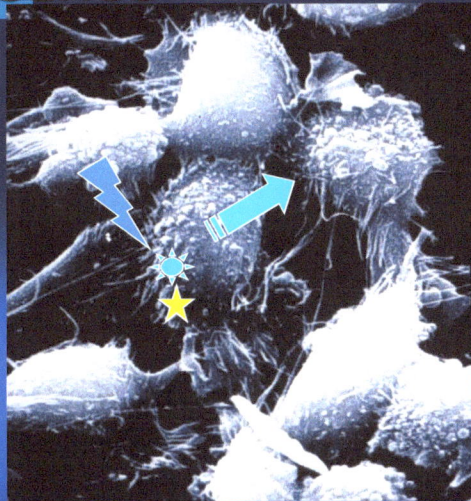

Dermatopathology Immunofluorescence

- **Antibodies are specific for proteins.**
- **Must be able to visualize.**
- **Fluorescein (FITC) gives off fluorescence under UV light.**

88

Figure 60. Scanning electron micrograph of cultured bladder tumor cells. The antibody (yellow star) attaches to the appropriate antigen (cell surface) and has a fluorescent label attached to it (blue sun). Upon excitation by UV light (lightning bolt) the label gives off apple green fluorescence (arrow).

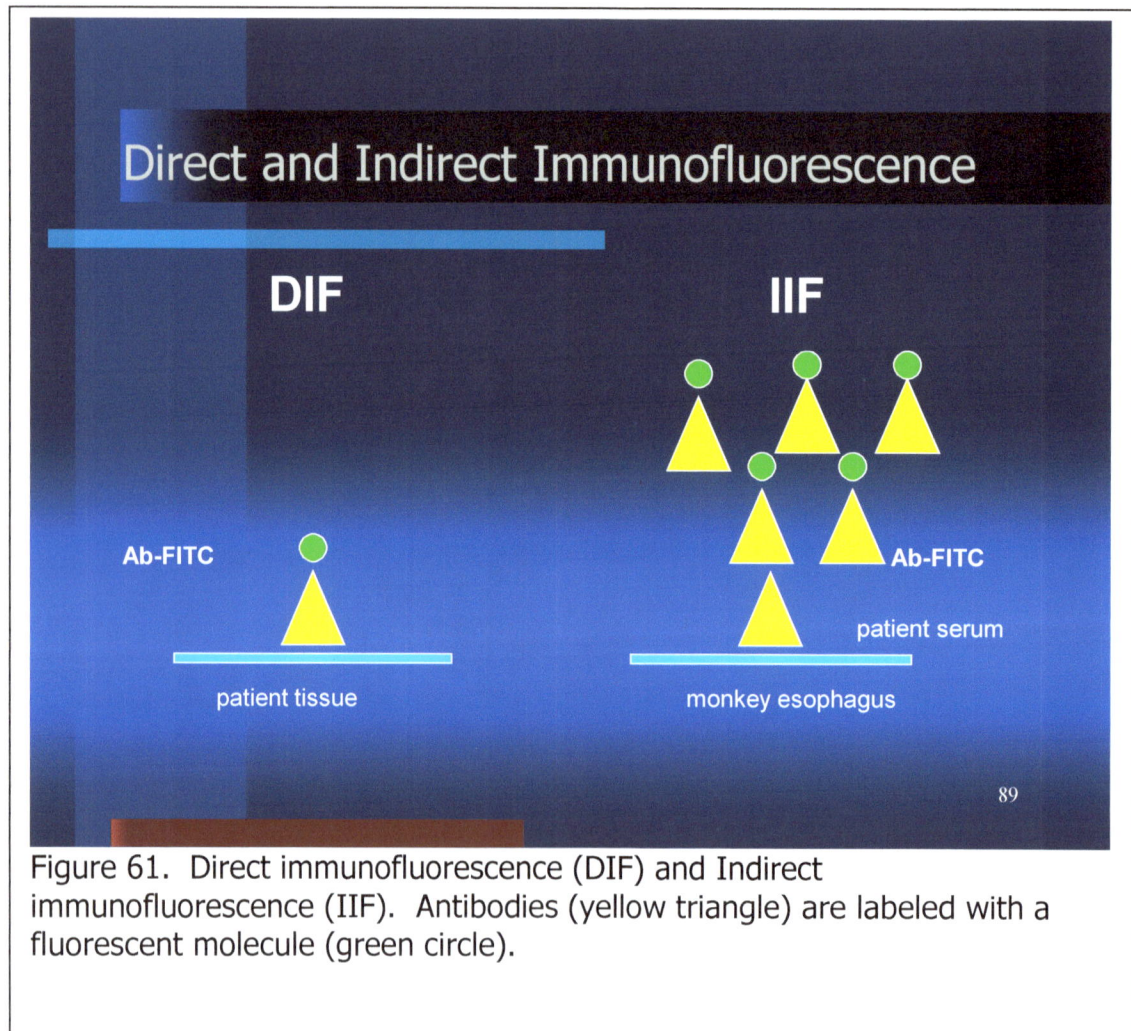

Figure 61. Direct immunofluorescence (DIF) and Indirect
immunofluorescence (IIF). Antibodies (yellow triangle) are labeled with a
fluorescent molecule (green circle).

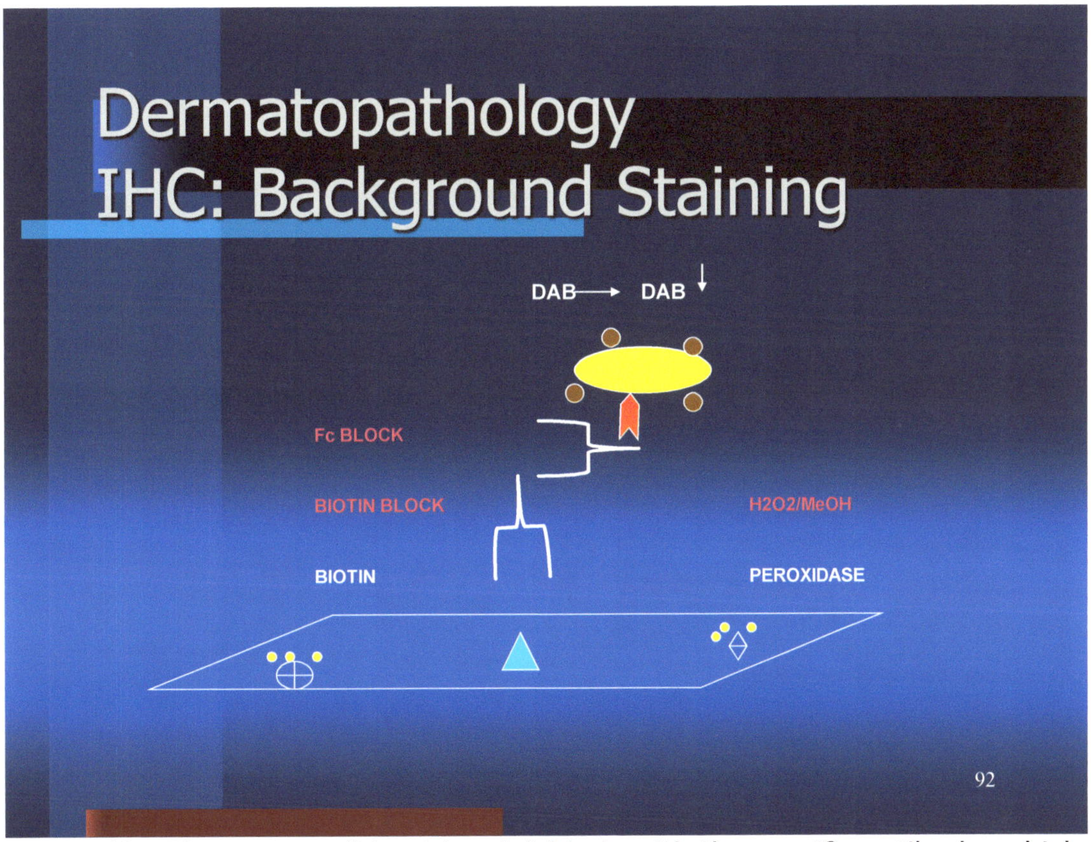

Figure 62. The antigen (blue triangle) binds with the specific antibody, which then can bind the secondary antibody, containing the link (red arrow). The final polymer/enzyme combination (yellow ellipse) binds to the link. Development of this combination results in the precipitation of the chromogen (DAB) at the site of antibody localization (brown circles). Ancillary reagents can block non-specific binding (i.e. hydrogen peroxide, biotin block, Fc block). Newer polymer methods overcome most of the non-specific background issues.

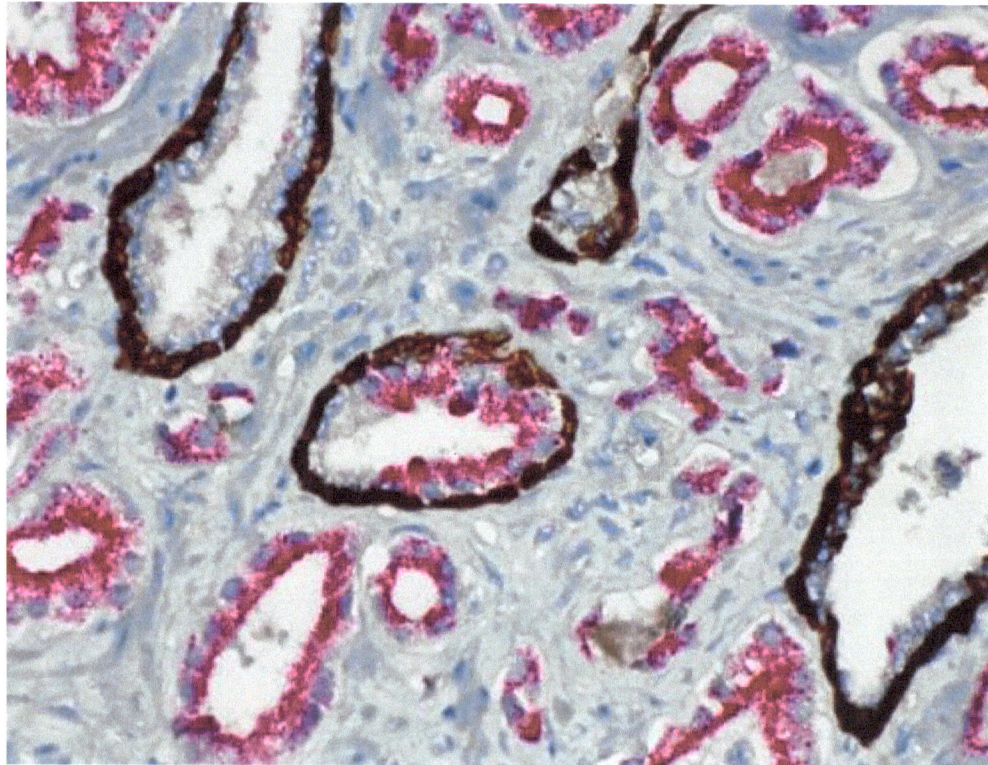

Figure 63. Prostate needle biopsy PIN4 staining by IHC method. Both red and brown chromogens are visualized.
Original magnification   x 600

Appendix

Procedure Section

HEADINGTON PROCEDURE FOR ALOPECIA / HAIR LOSS SPECIMENS

PRINCIPLE

Skin biopsies taken from the scalp may be for pathological diagnosis of alopecia (i.e. baldness, hair loss). It is important that the number of hair follicles can be measured. For this reason, skin specimens are prepared during the surgical gross in a particular way.

SPECIMEN

Skin specimens submitted for hair loss are almost always punch specimens.

PROCEDURE

1. When the requisition is reviewed, it should be brought to the attention of the grossing technician if any of the following terms are designated: "alopecia, hair thinning, hair loss, traction, baldness".
2. If this is the case, the grossing technician will split the punch specimen , parallel to the epidermis, as follows:

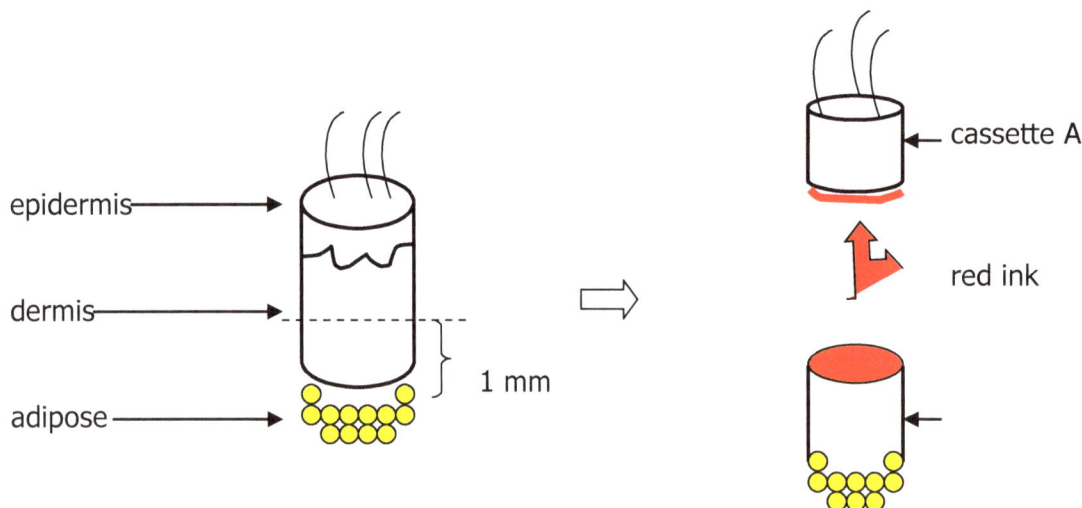

epidermis

dermis

adipose

1 mm

cassette A

red ink

3. The gross description will contain information that indicates that the "Headington" procedure was done.
4. The specimens will be embedded cut surface (i.e. red ink surface) down.

REFERENCE

Headington JT. Transverse microscopic anatomy of the human scalp. Arch Dermatol 1984; 120:449.

PROCEDURE FOR PREPARING NAIL SPECIMENS

PRINCIPLE

Toenail or fingernail specimens may be received in the laboratory with a differential diagnosis that may include fungal infection or melanoma, arising in the nail bed. This procedure describes how to fix the tissue and soften it such that it can be cut and stained with routine hematoxylin and eosin (H&E) and other special stains such as periodic acid Schiff's, Fontana-Masson and immunoperoxidase methods.

SPECIMEN

Fixation.   Nail specimens fixed in 10% neutral buffered formalin.

REAGENTS

Nail softener solution

Tween 85   5 ml
        [Sigma catalog # P4634]
10% formaldehyde   95 ml

CAUTION: Formaldehyde is toxic by inhalation and if swallowed. Irritating to the eyes, respiratory system, and skin. May cause sensitization by inhalation or skin contact. Risk of serious damage to eyes. May cause cancer. Repeated or prolonged exposure increases the risk. Wear safety glasses, chemical resistant gloves, and an apron. Work under a hood.

PROCEDURE

1. Confirm that the specimen is a nail either visually or from the requisition.
2. If the specimen is too large to fit into a cassette, cut into appropriate sizes and submit in multiple cassettes if necessary, such that all tissue is submitted.
3. Place the entire cassette(s) into the nail softening solution and allow to stand overnight.
4. Remove from the nail softening solution and place into formalin for later loading onto the tissue processor.
5. Process as usual, with at least an eight hour processing time.
6. Embed as usual with the nail pieces up on edge in the mold.
7. Once the sections are cut, they should be picked up on gelatin coated slides and baked in a conventional oven at 65 C for a minimum of 45 minutes. This will insure that the sections remain on the slide, regardless of the staining method.

REFERENCES

1. Rosai J. Ackerman's Surgical Pathology. 7th ed. CV Mosby, Washington DC, 1989. as modified by CM Chapman.

PROCEDURE FOR PREPARING GELATIN COATED SLIDES

PRINCIPLE

Certain specimens are received in the histology lab that require the sections to be picked up on specially coated slides. Decalcified bone and nail specimens should be picked up on gelatin coated slides.

SPECIMEN

Routinely processed, paraffin embedded blocks of decalcified bone and nail tissues.

REAGENTS

0.5% Gelatin solution
Gelatin	1.0 gm
[Fisher catalog # G8-500]	
Distilled water	200 ml

PROCEDURE

1. Add 1.0 gm of gelatin to 200 ml distilled water in a glass beaker that has been previously warmed on a hot plate to 60 C.
2. Allow to dissolve.
3. Transfer to a 250 ml plastic slide holder.
4. Load clean microscope slides into the vertical slide holder.
5. Immerse the slide racks containing the slides into the gelatin solution. Allow to soak for one minute.
6. Remove and allow to dry in the fume hood.
7. Place slides into storage boxes and keep in the refrigerator. This will inhibit bacterial growth. Use a one year expiration date.

REFERENCES

1. Bancroft JD ed. Theory and Practice of Histological Techniques. Churchill and Livingstone, 3rd edition, 1990, as modified by CM Chapman.

DECALCIFICATION OF BONE SPECIMENS

PRINCIPLE
Mineralized bone specimens may be received in the histology lab that require the specimens to be decalcified, such that they can be routinely processed and embedded in paraffin. Rather than a rapid decalcification with nitric or hydrochloric acid, this method employs a mixture of formic acid and formaldehyde. The formic acid is a weak acid that decalcifies slowly, but gently, and the formaldehyde allows fixation to continue while the decalcification takes place. The resulting histology is superior to other methods that use rapid decalcifiers.

SPECIMEN
Fixation: 10% formaldehyde (it is better to use non-buffered formula). Make certain that the bone is completely fixed prior to decalcifying.

REAGENTS
Decalcification solution
Formic acid	100 ml
10% formaldehyde	900 ml

CAUTION: Formaldehyde is toxic by inhalation and if swallowed. Irritating to the eyes, respiratory system, and skin. May cause sensitization by inhalation or skin contact. Risk of serious damage to eyes. May cause cancer. Repeated or prolonged exposure increases the risk. Wear safety glasses, chemical resistant gloves, and an apron. Work under a hood.
CAUTION: Formic acid is corrosive. Wear safety glasses, chemical resistant gloves, and an apron. Work under a hood. Always add acid last.

PROCEDURE
1. ***Determine that the specimen is bone, either visually or from the requisition.***
2. Make certain that the bone is already fixed completely. If it is not, transfer the bone to fresh formaldehyde fixative for 24 –48 hours, ideally using a shaker to keep the solution moving.
3. Once fixation is complete, transfer the bone specimen to the decalcification solution. Again, use agitation on a shaker if possible.
4. Pour off the solution and replace with fresh every 24 hours until the bone is completely decalcified. As the decalcification progresses, try to cut the specimen with a blade into smaller pieces. The resulting increased surface area will speed up the process.
5. When decalcification is complete, pour off the solution and rinse in running tap water for 1-2 hours.
6. Place the tissue in cassettes and process routinely into paraffin.
7. When sections are cut, pick them up on gelatin coated slides and bake in an oven at 60 C for a minimum of 45 minutes.

REFERENCES

1. Sheehan D. Theory and Practice of Histotechnology. 2nd ed. Chapter 6. CV Mosby, St. Louis, 1980, as modified by CM Chapman.

PROCEDURE FOR DETERMINING THE ENDPOINT OF DECALCIFICATION

page 1 of 1

PRINCIPLE

Mineralized bone specimens may be received in the histology lab that require the specimens to be decalcified, such that they can be routinely processed and embedded in paraffin. Whether employing rapid or slow decalcification techniques, it is important to determine the end point of the decalcification procedure.

SPECIMEN

Bone specimens that have undergone decalcification.

REAGENTS

5% ammonium hydroxide

Ammonium hydroxide, concentrated	5 ml
Distilled water	95 ml

5% ammonium oxalate

Ammonium oxalate	5 gm
Distilled water	100 ml

CAUTION: Ammonium hydroxide is corrosive. Wear safety glasses, chemical resistant gloves, and an apron. Work under a hood. Always add acid last.

PROCEDURE

1. Draw 5 ml of decalcifying solution, from the bottom of the container, which has been in contact with the tissue for 6-12 hours, and add to an empty beaker.
2. Add 5 ml each of 5% ammonium hydroxide and 5% ammonium oxalate.
3. Mix and let stand 15 minutes.
4. A cloudy solution caused by calcium oxalate indicates that the specimen is not thoroughly decalcified. Such a result indicates the necessity of changing the decalcifying solution and continuing the decalcification process.
5. When a milky solution is no longer obtained from such a mixture, the specimen is completely decalcified. The test can be performed as frequently as necessary.

REFERENCES

1. Luna L. ed. Manual of Histologic Staining Methods of the Armed Forces Institute of Pathology. 3rd ed., McGraw-Hill, New York, 1968, page 10.

PERIODIC ACID SCHIFF'S STAIN

PRINCIPLE

The Periodic acid-Schiff reaction (PAS) detects tissue carbohydrates, particularly for glycogen when used with a diastase digestion. Initial treatment of tissue sections with periodic acid cleaves the carbohydrate rings and produces aldehyde groups that subsequently react with Schiff reagent to produce bright pink coloration at the site of carbohydrate localization. Use of diastase digestion prior to the reaction will remove glycogen. This is important when attempting to localize fungi, whose cell walls are carbohydrate. Thus the PAS reaction can be used to localize both glycogen and fungi.

SPECIMEN

Fixation.   Formalin preferred. Other fixatives may be used.
Sectioning.   Cut paraffin sections at 5 microns.

QUALITY CONTROL

Include a known positive control with each run. Use skin (basement membrane), liver (glycogen) and/or fungal tissue cut at 5 microns for the control slide.

REAGENTS

Diastase/Amylase digestion solution (MAKE FRESH!)

Amylase   1.0 g
[Sigma catalog # 10070- alpha amylase from *Bacillus subtilis*]
0.02M Monobasic potassium phosphate   46.0 ml
0.02M Dibasic sodium phosphate   4.0 ml
[Alternatively, use phosphate buffered saline (PBS) from Polyscientific, catalog # S 2213]

0.02 M Monobasic potassium phosphate

Monobasic potassium phosphate   1.4 g
Distilled water   500 ml

0.02 M Dibasic sodium phosphate

Dibasic sodium phosphate   1.4 g
Distilled water   500 ml

1% Periodic Acid (MAKE FRESH!)

Periodic acid   1.0 g
Distilled water   100 ml
CAUTION: Periodic acid is corrosive. Wear safety glasses, chemical resistant gloves and an apron. Work under a hood. Always add acid last.

PERIODIC ACID SCHIFF STAIN

Schiff's Reagent

1. Purchase from Rowley Biochemical Institute (Product No. SO-429)

Store in refrigerator until expiration date.

2. Make as follows:

- boil 220 ml of distilled water
- add 1.0 g basic fuchsin
- let cool to 50 C
- add 20.0 ml of 1N HCl
- add 1.0 g anhydrous potassium metabisulfite
- store in refrigerator for 48 hours; solution should be straw colored
- add 2.0 g activated charcoal; mix well for 5 minutes
- filter through 2 layers of filter paper; the solution should be clear; if not, add more carbon and/or potassium metabisulfite
- store in refrigerator; stable for three months

CAUTION: Hydrochloric acid is corrosive. Wear safety glasses, chemical resistant gloves, and an apron. Work under a hood. Always add acid last.

0.5% Sodium Borate

Sodium borate	0.5 gm
Distilled water	100.0 ml

PROCEDURE

1. Deparaffinize and hydrate to distilled water.

FOR PAS+D

2. Place slides into amylase solution for 10 minutes at room temp. **MAKE FRESH!**

3. Wash well in running tap water for 7 rinses.

4. Proceed with step #5 below.

FOR PAS

5. 1% periodic acid for 10 minutes **MAKE FRESH!**

6. Wash well in running tap water for 7 rinses.

PERIODIC ACID SCHIFF STAIN

PROCEDURE (continued)

7. Schiff reagent for 10 minutes. <u>Pour the used solution into the special stains waste container.</u>

8. Rinse well in tap water for 3 changes.

9. Sodium borate for 1 minute; rinse in tap water for 3 changes.

10. Richard Allan hematoxylin I for 5 minutes.

11. Rinse in tap water

12. Bluing reagent for 10 seconds.

13. Rinse in tap water for 3 changes.

14. Dehydrate, clear and coverslip.

RESULTS

Fungi and glycogen..red/pink

Nuclei...blue

REFERENCES

1. Sheehan, Dezna C.: <u>Theory and Practice of Histotechnology.</u> Second edition. **9:** 164-166. Columbus: Batelle Press, 1980.
2. Lillie, RD and Fulmer, HM: <u>Histopathologic Technic and Practical Histology</u>, ed. 4, New York, 1976, McGraw-Hill Book Co.
3. McManus, JFA: The histological and histochemical uses of periodic acid. *Stain Technol*, **23**: 99-108, 1948, The Williams and Wilkins Co.
4. Luna, Lee (Editor): <u>Manual of Histologic Staining Methods of The Armed Forces Institute of Pathology.</u> Third edition. **10**: 158-160. New York: McGraw-Hill Book Company, 1968.
5. Mangan, VM et al: An amylase reagent with a long shelf life for the removal of glycogen from tissue sections. *J. Histotechnol.* **25**: 153-154, 2002.

PERIODIC ACID SCHIFF'S ON HAIR SHAFTS

page 1 of 1

PRINCIPLE: The periodic acid-Schiff reaction (PAS) detects tissue carbohydrates, particularly for glycogen when used with a diastase digestion. Use of diastase digestion prior to the reaction will remove glycogen. This is important when attempting to localize fungi, whose cell walls are carbohydrate. Thus the PAS reaction can be used to localize both glycogen and fungi. Fungi are detected both with, and without, diastase digestion.

SPECIMEN: Formalin preferred. Other fixatives may be used. 5 micron paraffin sections.

QUALITY CONTROL: Include a known positive control with fungal tissue.

PROCEDURE:
1. Confirm the number of hair shafts present in the specimen bottle.
2. Pour off the formalin fixative into a beaker.
3. Rinse with distilled water for 5 minutes.
4. Pour off into the waste beaker.
5. Add enough 0.5% periodic acid to cover the hair shafts.
6. Incubate for 10 minutes. Pour off into the waste beaker.
7. Rinse with distilled water for 5 minutes.
8. Add enough Schiff's reagent to cover the hair shafts.
9. Incubate for 20 minutes. Pour off into the waste beaker.
10. Rinse with distilled water for 2 minutes. Pour off into the waste beaker.
11. Rinse with tap water 3 times 3 minutes. Pour off into the waste beaker.
12. Leave specimen cap off and allow to air dry for 30 minutes.
13. Label a microscope slide with the accession number, patient name, PAS, and date.
14. Mount the hair shafts on the slide with Permount, and a cover glass.

RESULTS:
Fungi will appear as bright pink strands on the hair shaft, if present.

MASSON'S TRICHROME

PRINCIPLE

This method uses a sequence of procedures that use a nuclear stain and a plasma stain, followed by phosphomolybdic acid, then followed with a collagen fiber stain. This allows for a three-color stain differentiation of nuclei (black), collagen (blue) and muscle (red).

SPECIMEN

Fixation.   Formalin may be used; Bouin's is preferred. Tissues fixed in formalin may be mordanted in Bouin's solution, Gram's iodine or citrate buffer for one hour at 56 C or overnight at room temperature.

Sectioning.   Cut paraffin sections at 5 microns.

QUALITY CONTROL

Include a known positive control with each run. Sections of skin or intestine may be used.

REAGENTS
Weigert's iron hematoxylin solution

Solution A

Hematoxylin crystals	1.0 gm
Alcohol, 95%	100.0 ml

Solution B

Ferric Chloride, 29% aqueous	4.0 ml
Distilled water	95.0 ml
Hydrochloric acid, concentrated	1.0 ml

Working Solution **(MAKE FRESH!)**

Equal parts of solution A and B.
Not recommended for routine use. A very good and useful nuclear stain for special stains requiring hematoxylin.

CAUTION: Hydrochloric acid is corrosive. Wear safety glasses, chemical resistant gloves, and an apron. Work under a hood. Always add acid last.

Biebrich Scarlet

Biebrich scarlet	1.0 gm
Glacial acetic acid	1.0 ml
Distilled water	100.0 ml

1% Phosphomolybdic Acid

Phosphomolybdic acid	1.0 gm
Distilled water	100.0 ml

MASSON'S TRICHROME

REAGENTS (continued)

1.25% Aniline Blue Solution

Glacial acetic acid	4.0 ml
Distilled water	200.0 ml
Aniline blue	2.5 gm

1% Acetic Acid

Glacial acetic acid	1.0 ml
Distilled water	100.0 ml

CAUTION: Acetic acid is corrosive. Wear safety glasses, chemical resistant gloves, and an apron. Work under a hood. Always add acid last.

0.01 M Cit*rate Buffer*

0.15 M citric acid =	3.0 gm in 100 ml distilled water
0.1 M sodium citrate =	3.0 gm in 100 ml distilled water

Add equal parts of the above together to make citrate buffer pH 4.0. Adjust pH with sodium citrate to make citrate buffer at pH 6.0.
[Alternatively, use 0.01M citrate buffer pH 6.0 from PolyScientific, Bay Shore, NJ, catalog # S2307.]

Gram's Iodine

Iodine	1.0 gm
Potassium iodide	2.0 gm
Distilled water	300 ml

PROCEDURE

1. Deparaffinize and hydrate to distilled water.

2. Mordant formalin fixed tissue in Bouin's solution, Gram's iodine or citrate buffer pH 6.0 for 60 min at 56C.
[**Alternatively:** Run down, and mordant overnight at room temp.]

3. Rinse sections quickly in water.

4. Stain in Weigert's iron hematoxylin for 10 minutes. ***Make fresh right before use !*** Discard solution into special stains waste container.

MASSON'S TRICHROME

PROCEDURE (continued)

5. Wash in running tap water for 5 minutes.

6. Stain in Biebrich scarlet solution for 5 minutes. <u>Save solution.</u>

7. Rinse in distilled water, quickly.

8. Mordant in 1% phosphomolybdic acid for 2 minutes. <u>Save solution.</u>

9. Stain in aniline blue solution for 2 minutes. <u>Save solution.</u>

10. Rinse in water until no more color comes off of sections.

11. Rinse in 1% acetic acid solution for 1 minute.

12. Dehydrate, clear and coverslip.

RESULTS

Collagen .... intense blue
Nuclei .... blue to black
Cytoplasm, muscle fibers, keratin, intercellular fibers........... red

REFERENCES

1. J. Tech. Methods, 12:75, 1929.
2. Lillie, R.D.: <u>Histopathological Technic and Practical Histochemistry</u>. Third Ed. 1965. p.556.
3. Moore J: Citrate buffer alternative to picric acid for Masson Trichrome Stain. *The J Histotechnol* 19:341-342, 1996.
4. Yu Y and Chapman CM. Masson's Trichrome: Post Fixation Substitutes. *The J Histotechnol*, 26:131-134, 2003.

BROWN AND BRENN STAIN FOR BACTERIA

PRINCIPLE
The most informative routine stain for demonstrating bacteria in tissue sections is the Gram stain, and this technique differentiates the bacteria into Gram-positive and Gram-negative categories. Gram-positive fungal filaments of *Nocardia* and *Actinomyces* may also be shown.

The procedure involves the application of a crystal violet solution, followed by iodine mordant to form a lake dye. Both Gram-positive and Gram-negative cells are colored blue-black after these two steps. Decolorization is the third major step, and its purpose is to render the Gram-negative cells colorless while leaving the blue-black dye lake in the Gram-positive cells. The final major step is counterstaining with basic fuchsin, and the Gram-negative cells are dyed pink-red.

SPECIMEN
Fixation.   10% neutral buffered formalin; 2.5% buffered glutaraldehyde; or Helly's. Bouin's fixed tissues do not stain satisfactorily.
Sectioning.   Cut paraffin sections at 5 microns.

QUALITY CONTROL

Include a known positive control with each run. Use tissue with both Gram-negative and Gram-positive organisms cut at 5 microns for the control slide.

REAGENTS

Crystal Violet Solution, 1% Aqueous
Crystal violet	1.0 gm
Distilled water	100 ml

[Alternatively, use Rowley Biochemical Institute, Danvers, MA, Product No. S0-316.]

5% Sodium Bicarbonate Solution
Sodium bicarbonate (reagent grade)	5.0 gm
Distilled water	100.0 ml

Dissolve the sodium bicarbonate in the distilled water in a glass beaker, using a magnetic stirrer. Store in a glass bottle at room temperature for up to 1 year.

Crystal Violet-Sodium Bicarbonate Working Solution
Crystal violet solution, 1% aqueous	40.0 ml
5% sodium bicarbonate solution	8.0 ml

Combine just before use.

BROWN AND BRENN STAIN FOR BACTERIA

Gram's Iodine
Iodine (reagent grade)	1.0 gm
Potassium iodide (reagent grade)	2.0 gm
Distilled water	300.0 ml

Dissolve the potassium iodide in 3-4 ml of distilled water in a glass beaker, using a magnetic stirrer. Add the iodine and dissolve completely before adding the remaining amount of water. Store in a brown bottle at room temperature for up to 1 year.

Stock Basic Fuchsin Solution
Basic fuchsin (Color Index 42500)	0.25 gm
Distilled water	100.0 ml

Dissolve the basic fuchsin in the distilled water in a glass beaker, using a magnetic stirrer. Store in a glass bottle at room temperature for up to 1 year.

Working Basic Fuchsin Solution
Stock basic fuchsin solution	10.0 ml
Distilled water	100.0 ml

Combine the stock basic fuchsin solution and distilled water in a glass bottle. Store at room temperature for up to three months.

Gallego's Differentiating Solution
Distilled water	100.0 ml
Formalin, 37% to 40% (reagent grade)	2.0 ml
Glacial acetic acid (reagent grade)	1.0 ml

Combine the distilled water, formalin, and glacial acetic acid in a glass bottle. Store at room temperature for up to 1 month.

CAUTION: Formaldehyde is toxic by inhalation and if swallowed. Irritating to the eyes, respiratory system, and skin. May cause sensitization by inhalation or skin contact. Risk of serious damage to eyes. May cause cancer. Repeated or prolonged exposure increases the risk. Wear safety glasses, chemical resistant gloves, and an apron. Work under a hood.

CAUTION: Acetic acid is corrosive. Wear safety glasses, chemical resistant gloves, and an apron. Work under a hood. Always pour water into the container first, and then slowly add the acid.

BROWN AND BRENN STAIN FOR BACTERIA

0.1% Tartrazine

Tartrazine (Color Index 19140; Acid Yellow 23)	0.1 gm
Distilled water	100.0 ml
Glacial acetic acid (reagent grade)	0.2 ml

Dissolve the tartrazine in the distilled water in a glass beaker, using a magnetic stirrer. Add the glacial acetic acid. Store in a glass bottle at room temperature for up to 1 year.

CAUTION: Acetic acid is corrosive. Wear safety glasses, chemical resistant gloves, and an apron. Work under a hood. Always pour water into the container first, and then slowly add the acid.

Acetone (Histological Grade)

Fisher Scientific (Catalog No. A16P-4)
Store at room temperature in a flammable cabinet.

CAUTION: May cause liver and kidney damage. Do not breathe vapors; use with adequate ventilation. Wear safety glasses, chemical resistant gloves, and an apron.

Acetone:Xylene Mixture

Acetone, histologic grade	100.0 ml
Xylene, histologic grade	100.0 ml

Combine the acetone and xylene in a glass bottle. Store at room temperature for up to 1 year.

CAUTION: Acetone and xylene may cause liver and kidney damage. Do not breathe vapors; use with adequate ventilation. Wear safety glasses, chemical resistant gloves, and an apron. Work under a hood while preparing this mixture.

PROCEDURE

1. Deparaffinize and hydrate to distilled water.

2. Stain in crystal violet-sodium bicarbonate working solution for 1 minute. Pour the used solution into the special stains waste container.

3. Rinse in distilled water; shake off excess.

4. Mordant in Gram's iodine for 1 minute. Save solution.

5. Rinse in distilled water; shake off excess.

BROWN AND BRENN STAIN FOR BACTERIA

PROCEDURE: (continued)
6. Differentiate by dipping in acetone until blue color no longer streams away from the section (approximately 5-10 seconds). Pour the used acetone into the waste acetone container.

7. Quickly rinse in distilled water.

8. Stain in working basic fuchsin solution for 5 minutes. Save solution.

9. Wash in distilled water; shake off excess.

10. Differentiate and fix the basic fuchsin with Gallego's solution for 1 minute. Solution may be used for two weeks before being discarded in the special stain waste container.

11. Rinse thoroughly in distilled water. Blot slides slightly to remove excess water, but do not allow tissue to dry.

12. Dip in tartrazine for 10 seconds. Timing is critical. Immediately blot away excess, but not to dryness. Save solution.

13. Rinse quickly in acetone, then place in the acetone:xylene mixture. Pour the used solutions into the waste acetone container.

15. Clear in xylene and coverslip.

RESULTS
Gram-positive organisms... blue to blue-violet
Gram-negative organisms.. red
Nuclei... red
Other tissue elements... yellow

REFERENCES

1. Sheehan, Dezna C.: Theory and Practice of Histotechnology. Second edition. 13:   233-235. Columbus: Batelle Press, 1980.

VERHOEFF VAN GIESON STAIN FOR ELASTIC TISSUE

PRINCIPLE

The first step of this procedure uses a hematoxylin - ferric chloride - iodine solution to overstain the tissue section. Subsequent differentiation with dilute ferric chloride removes the stain from tissue elements, while leaving the elastic fibers and nuclei stained black. Van Gieson's is used as a counterstain and colors the collagen bright red and other tissue elements yellow.

SPECIMEN

Fixation.   Formalin or Zenker's (non-mercury recommended); any well-fixed tissue will work. It is not necessary to remove any mercury deposits since they will be removed by the staining solution.

Sectioning.   Cut paraffin sections at 5 microns.

QUALITY CONTROL

Include a known positive control with each run; skin is preferred.

REAGENTS

Verhoeff Stain
Hematoxylin	1.0 gm
Absolute alcohol	50 ml
10% ferric chloride	25 ml
Lugol's iodine	25 ml

Combine hematoxylin and alcohol in a small Erlenmeyer flask and dissolve with the aid of gentle heat. Filter and add the ferric chloride and Lugol's iodine.

Lugol's Iodine
Iodine	1.0 gm
Potassium iodide	2.0 gm
Distilled water	100 ml

10% Ferric Chloride
Ferric chloride	10.0 gm
Distilled water	100 ml

2% Ferric Chloride
10% ferric chloride	20 ml
Distilled water	80 ml

Van Gieson Solution
Saturated aqueous picric acid	100 ml
1% acid fuchsin, aqueous	5 ml

VERHOEFF VAN GIESON STAIN FOR ELASTIC TISSUE

PROCEDURE

1. Deparaffinize and hydrate to distilled water.

2. Immerse slides in Verhoeff stain for 15-60 minutes, or until completely black. Check after 15 minutes. Discard solution.

3. Rinse excess stain with distilled water.

4. Differentiate in 2% ferric chloride solution until background is gray to colorless and elastic fibers stand out black (i.e. three quick dips). Discard solution.

5. Rinse quickly in distilled water and check under the microscope.

6. Rinse in distilled water.

7. Rinse with 95% ethanol to remove iodine. Discard ethanol.

8. Rinse in distilled water for 5 minutes.

9. Counterstain with Van Gieson's solution for 2 minutes. Save solution.

10. Dehydrate, clear and coverslip.

RESULTS

Elastic fibers...	blue to black
Nuclei...	blue to black
Collagen...	red
Other tissue elements...........................	yellow

REFERENCES

1. Mallory, FB: Pathological Technique, New York, 1961.
2. Sheehan, DC: Theory and Practice of Histotechnology. Second edition. 10:196-197. Columbus: Batelle Press, 1980.

MELANIN REMOVAL

PRINCIPLE

Some tissues, especially skin specimens, contain excessive melanin pigment. This pigment may obscure the final results of many routine (i.e. H&E) and special stains. This method describes how to remove melanin pigment from tissue sections.

SPECIMEN

Fixation.   Any well fixed tissue will work.

Sectioning.   Cut paraffin sections at 5 microns.

QUALITY CONTROL

Include a known positive control with each run; skin is recommended.

REAGENTS
0.25% Potassium Permanganate
Potassium permanganate..............................   0.25 g
Distilled water..   100 ml

5% Oxalic Acid
Oxalic acid...   5.0 g
Distilled water..   100 ml

CAUTION: Oxalic acid is corrosive. Wear safety glasses, chemical resistant gloves, and an apron. Work under a hood. Always add acid last.

PROCEDURE

1. Deparaffinize and hydrate to water.

2. 0.25% potassium permanganate for 1 hour.

3. Rinse in distilled water.

4. 5% oxalic acid for 5 minutes.

5. Rinse in distilled water.

6. Stain as usual for H&E, or other selected stain.

7. Dehydrate, clear and coverslip

REFERENCES

1. AFIP Manual of Histologic Staining Methods. Luna, ed. Third Edition, McGraw-Hill 1968.

HEMATOXYLIN AND EOSIN (H&E) STAIN

page 1 of 1

PRINCIPLE: Hematoxylin stains nuclear material a dark blue, while the eosin stains cytoplasm and connective tissue varying shades of pink.

SOLUTIONS:
1. Harris' hematoxylin
2. Alcoholic Eosin – working solution
3. Clarifier (i.e. acid alcohol)
4. Bluing reagent (i.e. ammonium hydroxide)

PROCEDURE:
1. Cut paraffin sections 4-5 microns. Bake at 60 C for 45 minutes; allow to cool.

SOLUTION	TIME	NOTES
xylene	2 x 5 min	Removes paraffin
100% alcohol	2 x 2 min	Removes xylene
95% alcohol	1 x 2 min	Begins hydration
Running water	2 min	Hydrates
Hematoxylin	5 min	Stains nuclei and tissue
Running water	2 min	Removes excess
Clarifier	1 min	Removes hematoxylin from tissue
Running water	2 min	Stops clarifier action
Bluing reagent	1 min	Changes hematoxylin from red to blue with positive ions
Running water	2 min	Stops bluing action
95% alcohol	1 min	Readies for eosin
Eosin	1 min	Stains cytoplasm pink
95% alcohol	15 seconds	Differentiates eosin into 3 shades
100% alcohol	2 x 2 min	Dehydrates
Xylene	2 x 5 min	Readies for coverslip

REAGENTS

Clarifier:	tap water	2,600 ml
	100% alcohol	700 ml
	hydrochloric acid, conc	2.0 ml
Bluing	tap water	3,500 ml
	ammonium hydroxide, conc	1.5 ml

SILVER PRECIPITATE REMOVAL

PRINCIPLE

Sometimes during the course of performing a silver stain (i.e. Fontana-Masson, Warthin-Starry, Modified Steiner, Methenamine silver, reticulum, etc.) the silver solution may precipitate on the surface of the microscope slide in a non-specific manner. This procedure describes a method that can be used to remove non-specific silver precipitate.

SPECIMEN

Fixation.   Formalin fixation; avoid alcohol containing fixatives since alcohol dissolves argentaffin granules; any silver stain.

Sectioning.   Cut paraffin sections at 5 microns.

QUALITY CONTROL

Include a known positive control with each run. Use tissue with argentaffin containing cells, such as stomach, intestine and/or skin.

REAGENTS

1% Potassium Ferricyanide
Potassium ferricyanide	1.0 gm
Distilled water	100 ml

5% Sodium Thiosulfate
Sodium thiosulfate	5.0 gm
Distilled water	100.0 ml

Silver Removal Working Solution
1% Potassium ferricyanide	10 ml
5% Sodium thiosulfate	40 ml

CAUTION: Potassium ferricyanide is toxic. Wear safety glasses, chemical resistant gloves, and an apron. Work under a hood. Always pour the sodium thiosulfate into the container first, and then slowly add the potassium ferricyanide.

SILVER PRECIPITATE REMOVAL

PROCEDURE: Use chemically clean glassware.

2. If a microscope slide is covered with precipitated silver after the silver impregnation step it will appear either as black precipitate, or have a silver mirrored appearance.

3. Remove the slide from the silver solution and rinse in distilled water.

4. Immerse in the Silver Removal Working Solution for 10 min.

5. Rinse in distilled water.

6. Return the slide to a **fresh** preparation of the silver solution from which it came.

6. Continue the procedure.

RESULTS

The precipitated silver will be removed by the solution, rendering the slides clear. They can then be stained by the selected procedure.

REFERENCES

1. Sheehan: <u>Theory and Practice of Histotechnology.</u> Second edition.
15: 276-277. Columbus, Batelle Press, 1980.

References

Bancroft JD, Gamble M. *Theory and Practice of Histological Techniques.* 5th Ed New York, NY, Churchill -Livingstone, 2002.

Brown et al. *Uniform Labeling of Blocks and Slides in Surgical Pathology.* Guideline from the College of American Pathologists Pathology and Laboratory Quality Center and the National Society for Histotechnology. Arch Pathol Lab Med. Accepted for publication March 12, 2015.

Carson FL, Hladik C. *Histotechnology: A Self-Instructional Text.* 3rd Ed. Chicago, Ill ASCP Press; 2009.

Centers for Disease Control. www.cdc.org
Chapman CM. "The H&E Stain: Far From Routine." *Advance for Medical Professionals* April 2002.

Chapman CM. *Dermatopathology: A Guide for the Histologist.* Copyright 2003.

Chapman CM: "Dermatopathology: All Skin Specimens Are Not the Same." *Histologic:* Vol. XLIII No. 2, December 2010.

Chapman CM: "Barcoding and Dermatopathology." *Advance for Medical Laboratory Professionals:* Vol. 23 No 9, May 9, 2011.

Chapman CM: "Histology Hardball: Solutions for Hard Tissue." *Advance for Medical Laboratory Professionals:* Vol. 24 No2, February 20, 2012.

Chapman CM. Histology Study Group. Presented at Region I meeting, hosted by MaSH. 2014.

Chapman CM, Dimenstein IB. *Dermatopathology Laboratory Techniques.* CreateSpace / Amazon.com, 2016.

Dapson and Dapson. *Hazardous Materials in the Histopathology Laboratory.* Fourth Edition. Anatech Limited. 2005.

Dimenstein, IB. Technical Note published in the Journal of Histotechnology 2016. Vol. 39, No. 3, pages 76-80.

References
(continued)

Human Hair Atlas – Microscopic. www.swgmat.org

Laboratory Safety. NSH Self Assessment Booklet. 1ˢᵗ edition. page 33, 2004.

Lewin K, DeWit SA and Lawson R. "Softening techniques for nail biopsies." *Arch Dermatol*, 107(2):223-224, 1973.

Lillie RD & Fulmer HM. *Histologic Technique and Practical Histochemistry*. New York: McGraw-Hill, pp.52-53, 1976.

Lo and Fisher. "The melanoma revolution: From UV carcinogenesis to a new era in therapeutics." *Science.* Vol 346, Issue 6212, pp. 945-949. 21 November 2014.

Luna, Lee (Editor): *Manual of Histologic Staining Methods of the Armed Forces Institute of Pathology.* Third edition. New York: McGraw-Hill Book Company, 1968.

Luna, Lee (Editor): *Manual of Histologic Staining Methods of the Armed Forces Institute of Pathology.* Third edition. New York: McGraw-Hill Book Company, 1968. p39, as modified by CM Chapman

Margeson LM, Chapman CM: "The use of zinc formalin as a sensitizer in silver stains for spirochetes." *J Histotech*, 19:135-138, 1996.

Mayo Clinic Website. www.mayoclinic.org

Microorganisms website. http://www.microbiologybytes.com/iandi/6a.html

OSHA Bloodborne Pathogen Standard – Fact Sheet. www.osha.gov

Pearse AGE. *Histochemistry,* 4th ed. Vol 1.Baltimore, Williams & Wilkins Co., 1980.

Scher RK, Rich P, Pariser D, Elewski B. "The epidemiology, etiology, and pathophysiology of onychomycosis." *Semin Cutan Med Surg*. 2013 Jun;32, (Suppl 1):S2-4.

Yu Y, Chapman CM: "Masson trichrome stain: post fixation substitutes." *J Histotechnol*, 26:131-134, 2003.

Product References

Device for Uniform Sectioning. Dimenstein, Izak. Grossing Technology in Surgical Pathology.
http://grossing-technology.com/newsite/

HistoGel: A gel preparation for handling extremely small specimens and cell suspensions. Thermo Fisher Scientific.

Histowrap: Wrapping paper used for containing small specimens. Obex Industries.

Tween 85: Detergent solution for use in softening nails. Sigma Aldrich.

Kimberly Clark Fluid Shield Mask: Used for protection during grossing.

Davidson Marking Inks, for inking of margins.

Sakura FineTek: Paraform cassettes, Embedding gel

PolyScientific R&D: Harris' hematoxylin, Eosin

Source Medical Products: marking inks, grossing supplies

Epilogue

Throughout his career, the author has worked in, and contributed knowledge to, cancer research. Please know that a portion of the profits from the sale of this book will be donated to:

The Jimmy Fund, located at the Dana-Farber Cancer Institute in Boston, Massachusetts.

The Jimmy Fund started in 1948 when the Variety Children's Charity of New England and the Boston Braves baseball team joined forces to help a 12-year-old cancer patient dubbed "Jimmy."

The Jimmy Fund has been supported by the Boston Red Sox since its inception, and Ted Williams gave his time and support to the cause. When he started visiting children at the Dana-Farber in the 1950's, almost every child with cancer died. **Today, three out of four children with cancer survive.**
(http://www.dana-farber.org/).

It is the author's hope that the information contained in this book will contribute to the methods used in diagnosing and treating all types of cancer, and that your donation will contribute to curing cancer not only in children, but in all patients.

Thank you for purchasing this book. The author is dedicated to increasing learning opportunities and knowledge in the pathology and histology fields. Please feel free to contact the author with comments and suggestions at:

cmchapman100@gmail.com

www.ingramcontent.com/pod-product-compliance
Lightning Source LLC
Chambersburg PA
CBHW041720210326

41598CB00007B/725